Stroke
Promising Research that Could Change Your Life

Walter L. Kilcullen

ISBN: 1507826087
ISBN 13: 9781507826089
Library of Congress Control Number: 2015901981
CreateSpace Independent Publishing Platform
North Charleston, South Carolina

"We wish you strong health, endless optimism, borderless happiness and love."

From my Russian friends, Igor and Elena Bazilov

"I wish you enough sun to keep your attitude bright. I wish you enough rain to appreciate the sun. I wish you enough happiness to keep your spirit alive. I wish you enough pain so that the smallest joys seem big. I wish you enough gain to satisfy your wants. I wish you enough loss to make you appreciate your possessions. And I wish you enough hellos to get you through the goodbyes."

From my Russian friend, Dr. Natasha Fedosova

TABLE OF CONTENTS

PART III: AMAZING STROKE STORIES

INTRODUCTION

In November, 2013, I published a book entitled <u>Brain Injury: Living a Productive Life After a Stroke or Traumatic Brain Injury.</u> The purpose was to provide the readers with ideas and activities to enhance their lives after suffering a brain injury. I have written this second book for two reasons. First, in the 2013 book I had three chapters on research being done with the goal of reversing the effects suffered by brain injury survivors. In this book, I have updated this research. It is my hope that in the future, doctors will be able to restore movement to limbs after a brain injury. They may also be able to restore speech and cognition.

The second reason for writing this book is to offer additional ideas and information to help the survivor live a better life. As a mentor for brain injury survivors for the past fifteen years, I have offered some of these activities and ideas to my survivor friends.

I have no medical background or experience in treating brain injury. I am simply a mentor trying to improve the lives of the brain injury survivors that I work with. To write this book, I have researched existing articles and studies and cited my sources when appropriate. In some cases I interviewed doctors and other professionals to get opinions and to clarify research.

As in the first book, most of the chapters in this book were published in or will be published between November, 2013 and November, 2015 in strokenetwork.org, for which I am a staff writer. All of these chapters were revised and up-dated for this book.

And finally, like the first book, I have written this book in simple language eliminating most of the technical terms so that understanding is not difficult. Most important, all of the research in chapters one through four is on-going. It is important, therefore, that the reader follow this ongoing research so that progress can be followed which may have a profound effect on survivors.

Part I: Promising Research

Chapter 1: Repetitive Transcranial Magnetic Stimulation: Promising Research

"Man is not going to wait passively for millions of years before evolution offers him a better brain" Corneliu E. Giurgea (Romanian biologist and chemist)

Transcranial Magnetic Stimulation (TMS) is a non-invasive procedure using electromagnetic induction to stimulate specific areas to the brain. An electromagnet (coil) device is placed over a specific area of the skull where short pulses are administered that easily passes through the skull. Repetitive Transcranial Magnetic Stimulation (rTMS) involves multiple stimulations, delivered at a specific frequency for a specific duration. Most studies completed or in progress that consider TMS as a treatment use this method of TMS.

Studies and trials to test whether rTMS can improve hand, finger, and arm function after a stroke have been going on for at least twenty years. RTMS does show promise for stroke rehabilitation. Although it is not yet approved by the FDA as a treatment for stroke, several studies show positive results in improving motor skills. Ongoing studies being conducted by numerous researchers are still in progress.

What takes so long to tell if rTMS can improve or reverse the effects of a stroke on motor function? Research starts with all the variables involved for each study proposal. Then it must be approved by the sponsoring body, usually an affiliated hospital. Next, the research team must obtain funding. And finally, the research team must solicit recruits for the study. Typically there are three phases. Phase l is a safety study involving animals and/or a small human group. Phase II involves a human study lasting two or more years. Phase III involves a much larger human population often from various teams from several hospitals.

The real time comes from the variables involved. These include:

+ Age of the subjects
+ Severity of the damage or lesion from the stroke
+ Where to apply the rTMS; affected brain hemisphere or unaffected hemisphere
+ Low frequency rTMS (1Hz to 4Hz) versus high frequency (5Hz to 10Hz) [Hz = cycles/second]
+ Type of stroke (hemorrhagic versus ischemic)
+ Number and duration of rTMS treatments
+ rTMS alone or combined with various manual therapies

All of these variables must be tested to draw conclusions as to the effectiveness of rTMS to treat motor deficits after a stroke.

There are close to 100 studies testing rTMS for stroke rehabilitation. These include completed studies, studies in progress, and planned studies. The large majority of studies in all three categories are designed for upper limb (hand, finger and/or arm) motor function. There are, however, a significant number of studies to treat aphasia after a stroke. I describe a few of these aphasia studies in Chapter 3. I read more than forty studies and I decided that I would summarize a few successful completed studies, a few studies in progress, and a few planned studies aimed at upper extremity function.

It is my hope that readers of this chapter who suffer from upper limb weakness or paralysis will follow studies that are ongoing or participate in a study that is planned. A list of studies planned or in progress can be found at clinicaltrials.gov. and new studies appear frequently.

Selected completed studies:
<u>Study:</u> "Low-Frequency TMS to Enhance Motor Recovery in the Sub-acute Phase After a Stroke." Conforto, Adriana, MD, PhD; Neurostimulation Laboratory, University of Sao Paulo, Sao Paulo, Brazil.

Study completed May, 2014
Low-frequency (1Hz) rTMS was delivered to the unaffected brain hemisphere, once per day for ten

days. Thirty subjects participated. Half were given the rTMS treatment, the other half were given sham (fake) rTMS treatment. All subjects had moderate to severe upper limb impairment and were less than forty five days post stroke as treatment began. Conclusion: I contacted Dr. Adriana Conforto to ask her about the study. She stated, "The study we did with rTMS to improve upper limb motor improvement suggested the inhibition of the unaffected hemisphere by low-frequency rTMS may be beneficial to enhance motor function of the paretic (partially paralyzed) upper limb, particularly in patients more severely affected. However, results from this proof-of-principal study were preliminary. Larger trials are necessary to check whether this intervention may be clinically useful."

I asked Dr. Conforto if she believed that it will be possible in the future to reverse or improve hand and arm paralysis even years post stroke. She answered, "I think it will be possible to improve function, and perhaps to find new ways to control a paretic limb, maybe not in all patients, but in many."

Study: "Primed vs. Unprimed rTMS in Chronic Stroke." Jessica M. Cassidy, PhD candidate, DPT, James R. Carey, PhD, P.T., Program in Physical Therapy and Rehabilitation Science, Clinical and Translational Science Institute, University of Minnesota, Minneapolis, Minnesota.

Study completed August, 2014 (results pending) Priming is an extra session of rTMS stimulation given before the delivery of low-frequency rTMS. The lab previously demonstrated the safety of 6 Hz priming with low-frequency rTMS in both adults and children. This study examined three priming/rTMS interventions in eleven adults over the age of eighteen with chronic (long standing) loss of function from stroke. All eleven participants received all three interventions in randomized order. Treatments included: 1. Ten minutes of real 6 Hz priming followed by ten minutes of low-frequency rTMS; 2. Ten minutes of sham (fake) 6 Hz priming followed by ten minutes of low-frequency rTMS; and, 3. Ten minutes of low-frequency priming followed by another ten minutes of low-frequency rTMS. All treatments were applied to the non-stroke side of the brain. Each week, participants completed two pre-tests and three post-tests to examine potential changes in motor function and cortical excitability in the stroke side of the brain. After each week of testing and treatment, participants took a one-week rest break before crossing over to receive the remaining interventions.

Conclusion: Results of the study are pending. I interviewed Jessica Cassidy, one of the investigators of this study. She stated, "I remain skeptical that we will be able to completely reverse arm and hand paralysis; however, I remain hopeful and driven to explore the capabilities of rTMS as an adjunct (supplement) intervention to traditional physical and occupational therapies to potentiate arm and hand movement."

Study: "Primed Low-Frequency rTMS and Constraint Induced Movement Therapy in Pediatric Hemiparesis: A Random Controlled Trial." Bernadette T. Gillick MD, PhD et. al., Department of Physical Medicine and Rehabilitation, University of Minnesota, Minneapolis, Minnesota.

Study completed 2013

Note: Hemiparesis means weakness on one side of the body. Constraint Induced Movement

Therapy is a therapy used in patients with paretic (partially paralyzed) hand and/or arm motor function. The patient wears a mitt (or splint, sling or other device) on the unaffected hand for a designated time for a designated number of days, weeks, or months. This forces the patient to use the affected limb. By having the patient engage in repetitive exercises using the affected limb the brain grows new neural pathways. This is called neuroplasticity.

Nineteen children (ten males, nine females) with congenital hemiparesis in an upper limb, between the ages of eight and seventeen (average age 10.8) were used for the study. Ten of the subjects were given five sessions of low-frequency rTMS alternating daily with CIMT. The nine remaining subjects received the same therapy except that the rTMS was sham (fake).
Conclusion: Results of the study included accepted professional tests to measure improvement in the affected upper limb. All participants finished the study with no adverse effects. Eight of the ten rTMS group showed significant motor improvement while only two out of nine

in the sham group showed significant improvement. More studies with larger populations are recommended.

I spoke to Dr. Gillick on the phone in September, 2014. She stated, "It is very possible in the future that rTMS combined with other more traditional therapies, such as physical therapy, occupational therapy, or CIMT, will improve upper limb function in stroke survivors with impaired function."

Recently, Dr. Gillick received a grant to study Transcranial Direct Current Stimulation (TDCS) as a treatment for stroke survivors with upper limb impairment. TDCS is similar to rTMS but it is delivered by two small 9 volt batteries rather than by magnetic coils. It is much less expensive than rTMS and it is hoped that it will deliver equal or better results than rTMS.

I asked Gr. Gillick if she thought that rTMS or TDCS will be able to improve upper limb function in ten years or less from now. She answered, "Neither. I see the use of these therapies as a stepping stone. In ten years I believe there will be new therapies including Laser Therapy and Implantable Devices."

Study "Effects of rTMS on Motor Functions in Patients with Stroke." Hsu, Wan-Yu, et. al., Institute of Brain Science, National Yang-Ming University, Taipei, Taiwan.

Study completed in 2013

This study analyzed control trials between 1990 – 2011.The studies analyzed 392 patients from thirty-four selected studies using rTMS to improve upper limb motor function (in other words, this is a study analyzing other studies). Conclusion: rTMS had a positive effect on motor function. Low frequency rTMS over the unaffected brain hemisphere may be more beneficial than high frequency rTMS over the unaffected brain hemisphere. Further studies using a larger patient population are needed to test various methods of using rTMS for improved upper limb motor function after a stroke.

Dr. Carolyn Patten PhD, Neurology and Dr. William Triggs MD, both researchers at the University of Florida and VA Brain Rehabilitation Research Center in Gainesville, Florida have been involved in several studies and have reviewed studies done by other researchers investigating the use of rTMS on motor dysfunction after stroke.

I was able to reach both doctors via e-mail in early 2013. Dr. Triggs stated, "rTMS as a treatment for stroke has potential, particularly when combined with physical or occupational therapy. However, more double blind studies using larger populations are needed before a definite conclusion can be reached."

Dr. Patten also responded and emphasized this point. "While we have not cracked the code, there is reason for optimism. There is a lot of work to be done. I hope that people who have experienced stroke will remain open to the idea, and that their health care providers will remain open to the idea so that all the labs investigating rTMS are able to do their studies and collectively we are able to advance knowledge and improve stroke rehabilitation."

Selected studies in Progress:
<u>Study:</u> "Efficiency and Safety Study of rTMS for Upper Extremity Motor Function Recovery

in Ischemic Stroke Patients." Paik, Nam-Jong, Seoul National University Bundang Hospital, Seoul, South Korea.

Expected completion: March, 2016

This study included forty subjects between ages twenty and eighty within ninety days or less post ischemic (clot) stroke. Half of the subjects received ten sessions of low-frequency (1Hz) rTMS over the primary hemisphere of the dominant hand. The other half received sham (fake) rTMS also in the same ten sessions. The goal is to improve upper extremity motor function.

Conclusion: I contacted Dr. Paik via e-mail. He states, "We hope that rTMS can facilitate motor recovery for the upper limb in subacute phase of stroke patients. There have already been some reports of positive effects in chronic (indefinite duration) stroke patients."

Study: "rTMS Study to Improve Functional Performance for Patients with Stroke." Lin, Yen-Nung, Taipei Medical University, Wan Fang Hospital, Taipei, Taiwan.

Expected completion January 2016

This study is to focus on motor function of the lower extremities. Sixty subjects from ages eighteen to eighty will receive low frequency (1Hz) rTMS for fifteen minutes followed by forty-five minutes of physical therapy for fifteen consecutive week-days. The goal is to improve lower extremity gait and function.

I was able to reach Dr. Lin by e-mail. I asked him if he thought it is possible in the future for rTMS treatment to reverse, or at least improve motor function in the upper extremities, even years post stroke. He said, "I know that many people including researchers view rTMS as a new hope for stroke treatment. Some published articles have shown rTMS to be effective in improving motor functions even for chronic stroke patients. However, the results from clinical trials are not consistent. Currently I think the evidence is not sufficient to make me believe that rTMS can improve motor function in upper extremities."

Note: This is the only study I found testing lower extremities. Dr. Lin's quote pertains to upper extremity studies.

Selected planned studies:
Study: "rTMS Use in Acute Stroke"
Principal investigator: James R. Carey, PhD; University of Minnesota Clinical Translational and Science Institute
Aim: Using rTMS to determine safety and to measure hand function improvement.

Study " Effects of rTMS Combined with Fluoxetine on Motor Recovery in Stroke Patients"; Principal investigator: Felipe Fregni, MD, PhD; Spaulding Rehabilitation Hospital, Charlestown, Massachusetts
Aim: To measure safety and efficiency of motor function combining rTMS and the drug Fluoxetine (Fluoxetine is used for depression; trade name is Prozac).

Study: "RTMS in Patients with Hemiplegic Stroke;" Principal Investigator: Suk Yun Kang, MD; Dongtan Sacred Heart Hospital, Republic of Korea.
Note: Dystonia is a disorder causing repetitive twisting movements resembling tremors of the affected body part(s). Note: hemiplegic means total paralysis in the arm, leg, or trunk
Aim: To investigate therapeutic effect on motor recovery in hemiplegic stroke using rTMS.

Study: "RTMS and Occupational Therapy in Children and Adults with Chronic Hemiparesis;" Principal investigator: Steve W. Wu, MD; Children's Hospital Medical Center, Cincinnati, Ohio
Aim: To determine if rTMS can augment occupational therapy in improving motor function in children (under ten) and young adults (under twenty one) with chronic hemiparesis
Note: Hemiparesis means weakness on one side of the body.

Study: "TMS for Focal Hand Dystonia;" Principal investigator: Rainer W Paine, MD; National Institute of Neurological Disorders and Stroke (NINDS), National Institute of Health Clinical Center, Bethesda, Maryland
Aim: To determine if rTMS can improve dystonia.

Readers should follow these and more future studies on clinicaltrials.gov.

Conclusions:

1. Using rTMS to improve motor control and function of the upper extremities shows promise for improvement after a stroke.

2. Using rTMS to improve motor function is more successful in patients whose stroke occurred within a few months. Most, but not all of the research studies were conducted with patients less than four months post stroke. It is probable that the shorter length of time that elapses before treatment, the better the outcome.

3. A majority of the studies showed an improvement in motor function after treatment with rTMS. However, there were some studies where no improvement occurred.

4. Adverse effects in all of the studies I looked at were either minor or were nonexistent.

5. It is clear that rTMS is more successful when combined with physical therapy, occupational therapy, or constraint induced movement therapy.

6. It is clear that rTMS treatment is more successful when a patient has hemiparesis (weakness but not paralysis) or paretic (partial paralysis) rather than hemiplegic (total paralysis).

7. Research is still in the early stages and FDA approval for using treatment for upper limb motor function after stroke is probably years away.

Chapter 2: Stem Cell Therapy: Promising Research

"A man should keep his little brain attic stocked with all the furniture that he is likely to use, and the rest he can put away in the lumber room of his library, where he can get it if he wants it" Arthur Conan Doyle (author and creator of Sherlock Holmes)

About eight years ago research being done using stem cells for stroke recovery centered on safety using rats as subjects.

I wrote an article for strokenetwork.org in November, 2012, based on updated research that was largely still using rats, but a few safety studies were using small groups of human subjects. Researchers were cautiously optimistic that someday stem cell therapy could be used to reverse or at least improve limb disabilities as a result of a stroke. That optimism continues today.

Most of the studies that I read while doing research for this chapter, and there were many, are using small groups of human subjects with safety being the primary measure and improved movement function being the secondary measure. This is a big step toward the goal of using stem cell therapy to treat weakness and paralysis in limbs as a result of a stroke.

Still, there are several obstacles to overcome:

+ deciding on the type of stem cells to be used, the dosage to be used, and the frequency and length of treatment
+ deciding what type of patient would benefit most: ischemic vs. hemorrhagic; recent stroke vs. chronic stroke; young vs. old survivors
+ deciding where to deliver the cells: intravenously vs. directly into the brain

Stem Cells: A stem cell is a cell in the human body that has the ability to grow other types of cells, as well as to self-renew. Depending on where they come from, how they are raised, and to what materials they are exposed, a stem cell may be coaxed to produce specific compounds or to differentiate into other specific cells. In almost all of the studies, past and present, that I read, researchers used or are using one of three types of stem cells.

Embryonic Stem Cells: When a woman's eggs are fertilized, the earliest cells of the embryo are stem cells. These are considered to be the most useful type of stem cells because they are "pluripotent", meaning that they theoretically have the ability to differentiate into any other cell type in the human body. Often these stem cells come from an embryo donated by the woman for research purposes. The use of embryonic stem cells for research studies is controversial because many people, led by religious groups, consider an embryo the beginning of life. In order to obtain the stem cells, the embryo is destroyed.

Umbilical Cord Stem Cells: Stem cells can also come from a baby's umbilical cord blood shortly after giving birth. These cells are increasingly being harvested and stored by families for possible use in the future should someone in the family require a stem cell transplant. They are now widely used in stroke recovery research.

Bone Marrow Stem Cells: Stem cells can also be derived from either the patient's own bone marrow or from a donor. If taken from the patient, it has the added benefit of not being rejected by the patient's body. Even though they come from bone marrow, these cells can also be made to become multiple other types of cells, such as nervous system cells.

There are many studies either completed or in progress so I chose three of the most recent studies to show the status of stem cell therapy for stroke rehabilitation. All of these studies have safety as a primary measurement and improved movement function as a secondary measurement.

Study: "A Study of Modified Stem Cell in Stable Ischemic Stroke." Principal Investigators: Gary K. Steinberg M.D., PhD, Stanford University School of Medicine; Joshua M. Rosenow M.D., Northwestern University Feinberg School of Medicine, et. al., 2014.

Study completed in 2014

Eighteen participants between the ages of eighteen and seventy-five, and between six and sixty months post stroke, were treated with a modified stem cell product taken from donated bone marrow stem cells. Each group of six was given a different dose stem cell product. Group one received 2.5 million; group two received 5.0 million; and group three received 10 million. The delivery method was by injecting the stem cells directly into the brain into several locations around the stroke lesion. The cells used in this study were treated to make them release a combination of compounds thought to help preserve cell function. The theory is that there are areas around a stroke location that are not functioning optimally and may be salvageable. It is hoped that the compounds secreted by these cells would encourage repair and renewal in these regions.

All eighteen patients saw some improvement in weakness or paralysis six months after treatment was completed. Two of the patients experienced dramatic improvement immediately after treatment. All eighteen patients will be followed until May, 2015 when the study is completed.

Brenda Goodman wrote an article about this study for <u>WebMD</u> entitled, "Stem Cells Show Promise for Stroke Recovery." (April 7, 2014). She quotes Dr. Gary K. Steinberg, a principal investigator of the study who said, "We had two patients who showed remarkable recovery. Both were women. They were very disabled. One was seventy-one and the other was thirty-three. The seventy-one year old could only move her left thumb. She could not move her arm or hand and could barely get her leg off the bed." He added, "The day after the surgery, she was lifting her arm over her head, and lifting her leg off the bed. She is walking now. She was wheelchair bound before."

Dr. Steinberg further stated, "Similarly, the thirty-three year old had a severe speech deficit and had trouble lifting her arm over her head. A year later her gait and speech have improved." Dr. Steinberg cautioned, "These types of recoveries are not typical….but we thought the circuits were dead. Now we know they are still viable. We just have to know how to activate them."

to benefit. The improvements we saw in these patients are very encouraging, but it is too early to draw definite conclusions. We need to do more tests to work out the dose and timescale for treatment before starting larger trials."

Professor Nagy Habib, also a principal investigator of the study, stated, "These are early but exciting data worth pursuing….our aim is to develop a drug based on the factors secreted by stem cells that could be stored in the hospital pharmacy so it could be administered to the patient immediately following diagnosis in the emergency room."

Study: "Pilot Investigation of Stem Cells in Stroke (PISCES I)," Principal Investigator: Keith Muir M.D., Glasgow Southern General Hospital, Glasgow, United Kingdom.

Study is ongoing

(PISCES I) Eleven male patients between the ages of sixty and eighty five, and between six months and five years post ischemic stroke, were given fetal stem cells at one of four doses (two million; five million; ten million; and finally twenty million) to measure safety and tolerance.

The stem cells were injected directly into the brain with the patient under anesthesia.

Each patient was followed for two years. Five of the first six patients showed improvement in function with no cell related adverse effects. There is no data yet on the final five patients treated. Although the primary aim of this study is to evaluate safety and tolerance of the stem cells, a secondary aim is to measure increase of function of the arm and hand. Each patient will have six scheduled appointments to the clinic for monitoring adverse effects and for neuro-functional testing during this follow-up two year period. The study is just concluding (March, 2015) and full results will be published soon.

A second study (PISCES II) is now recruiting patients. It will start with twenty subjects and, depending on initial analysis, will recruit up to forty one patients. To be eligible to partici-pate, a patient must have no useful function of the affected arm and hand at both twenty eight days and fifty six days post ischemic stroke, and be between the ages of forty and eighty nine. Although safety will still be monitored, there is more emphasis on function than there was with PISCES I.

The study involves giving each patient twenty million stem cells delivered directly into the brain. The purpose of the study is to determine if giving this dose of stem cells is likely to improve recovery in the affected arm and hand. If there is significant improvement in at least two patients out of the first twenty treated, the final twenty-one patients will be treated. The ultimate goal is to study large groups of patients in a PISCES III study but that will only happen if PISCES II is successful.

I contacted Dr. Muir via e-mail and he informed me that although no cell-related safety issues have surfaced so far, adverse effects may become evident in the years to come. In addition, he stated, "Some improvement in function was seen in the majority of trial patients; however, this cannot be attributed to cell therapy as we did not have a control group in the trial."

Conclusions: Optimism

+ Optimism for stem cell therapy to treat stroke continues to grow but there is still much to be done before any conclusions can be made about the effectiveness of stem cells as a treatment for stroke.

+ All of the studies that I read involved ischemic stroke which make up 80% to 87% of strokes. None of the studies involved stroke survivors who suffered a hemorrhagic stroke.

+ It is important for stroke survivors to follow studies that may change their lives in the future.

Chapter 3: Aphasia: Promising Research

"The important thing in science is not so much to obtain new facts as to discover new ways of thinking about them" Sir William Lawrence Bragg (British physicist)

Aphasia is defined as the loss of the ability to speak or understand language. About one in four stroke survivors experience some form of aphasia. It often occurs after a left brain stroke with varying degrees of severity and varying characteristics. There are many aspects of aphasia, but to keep it simple it is best to divide the term into "expressive aphasia," which means that patients have difficulty speaking and writing, and "receptive aphasia," which means that patients have difficulty understanding what is said to them, and difficulty reading. Some survivors have both.

I have been mentoring patients with aphasia for many years. One survivor that I mentor is unable to speak in sentences and is unable to express what she wants to say. Another speaks so rapidly that understanding what is said is very difficult. Another struggles with every word trying to express his thoughts. Symptoms may include:

+ difficulty in pronouncing or forming words
+ difficulty understanding or comprehending language
+ difficulty with or inability to read and/or write
+ a tendency to repeat words or phrases
+ difficulty or inability to use complete sentences
+ difficulty or inability to repeat words or phrases
+ poor enunciation
+ difficulty or inability to name objects

After a stroke occurs, the patient with aphasia will receive daily speech therapy to help in regaining as much language as possible. Very seldom does this result in complete recovery from aphasia. After being discharged from the hospital, survivors must try to improve on their own. I recommend the following:

Join a support group specifically for aphasia. Go to the National Aphasia Association web-site (www.aphasia.org) to find a support group nearest you. Scroll down to "aphasia community groups." Support groups are a great source to learn the latest research, ideas shared by other members, and for meeting friends with similar problems. If there is no aphasia support group near you, you can start your own. The NAA web-site tells you how.

Investigate available computer software and speech devices to see if they meet some of your needs. Bungalow Software, Parrott Software, Communication Scripts, Lumosity, and Lingraphica are examples.

Investigate clinics and community groups that specialize in aphasia. The NAA web site can help. Scroll down to "Aphasia Community" and then to "Aphasia Programs and Centers." This will enable you to see what is available near you.

Promising Research: Hope for the Future: Constraint Induced Aphasia Therapy (CIAT):

Also called Constraint Induced Language Therapy (CILT), or Intensive Language Action Therapy (ILAT): This treatment focuses on speech production, and the patient may only communicate by talking. The therapist uses many of the techniques used in conventional speech or language therapy, but the difference is in the intensity and the time per session. Between two and four hours per day is typical. Many studies using CIAT have been completed or are in progress. Below are two such studies and one review.

Study: "Constraint Induced Language Therapy in Early Aphasia Rehabilitation," Melanie Kirmess, PhD, Speech-Language Pathologist, Department of Special Needs Education, University Oslo, Norway; and Lynn M. Maher, PhD, Speech-Language Pathologist, University of Houston, Houston, Texas. Aphasiology, 24(6-8), June, 2010, pp. 725-736.

Study completed 2010
Three patients, one to two months post stroke, received CIAT for three hours per day for ten

days over a period of one to two months. Therapy included flash card activities using various frequency at four levels of difficulty, either in a small group or one-to-one with a trained speech language pathologist. Based on the card game activity, there is a correlation to effects on comprehension as well. You cannot speak or answer without understanding (at least parts) of the question.

Results: An overall improvement on language assessment tests was obtained. This was especially true for improvement on expressive speech tasks. Researchers concluded that further studies are warranted using larger populations.

I was able to reach Dr. Kirmess via email and asked her about the future of CILT in treating aphasia. She stated, "Our rehabilitation hospital, Sunnaas, includes regularly chronic stroke survivors in CILT groups, and we have positive outcome results for the majority, even years after the stroke. However, changes may only be seen on language tests, and not in everyday communication, or vice versa due to the heterogeneity of the persons attending, their severity of aphasia, and other personal/environmental factors. We so far do not know about the long term maintenance of those results, but are continuously investigating further studies"

Dr. Kirmess informed me about another program that she is heading called the SunCIST Program. This program with results was presented to the Academy of Aphasia Conference in San Francisco, California in 2012. The program provides groups of six aphasia patients ranging from mild to severe aphasia with three weeks (fifteen week-days) of inpatient intervention focusing on psychosocial and physical aspects, as well as use of language skills in natural social situations. The treatment includes CILT card game activities using high and low frequency stimuli with communicative relevance at various levels of complexity. CILT is applied in a small group of three participants and one by a trained Speech-Language Pathologist. Overall, each participant in the SunCIST program receives about forty-five hours of structured language activities as well as thirty hours of other group activities.

All participants completed a recognized standard assessment on the first and last day of the SunCIST program. At the time of the presentation to the Academy of Aphasia, despite a large variation in aphasia severity, all forty-six patients with chronic aphasia showed improvement in at least one subtest. Researchers believe that by continuing the SunCIST program, more data will become available to analyze the effectiveness of this approach in treating aphasia.

This presentation was also published: "The SunCIST Program – a Clinical Approach for Intensive Aphasia Rehabilitation," Kirmess, Melanie; Becker, Frank; Hvistendahl, Anne Katherine; Gunther, Live. Procedia – Social and Behavioral Sciences, 2012, Vol. 61, 18-19.

Study: "An Enhanced Protocol of CIAT II: A Case Series," Edward Taub, PhD, et. al., University of Alabama Birmingham, American Journal of Speech-Language Pathology, Vol. 23: 60-72, February, 2014. In this study, an expanded and enhanced form of the earlier version of CIAT is described; it is called CIAT II.

Study is ongoing

Whereas CIAT used a single exercise to improve language and speech, CIAT II is a more intense multi faceted approach. The study included four patients who suffered from moderate expressive aphasia after a stroke. Treatment was carried out for three and one half hours a day for fifteen consecutive week-days. It included (1) intensive training by a behavior method called "shaping" using a number of extensive language exercises in addition to a single original language card game. (2) strong discouragement of patient attempts to use gestures or other non-verbal means of communications. (3) a transfer package of behavioral techniques to promote transfer of treatment gains from the laboratory to real-life situations.

Results: Participation in speech in life situations improved significantly. In fact, positive results were ten times greater than the previous CIAT study. I was able to reach Dr. Taub via e-mail and asked him about the future of CIAT for aphasia rehabilitation. He stated, "The results suggest in preliminary fashion that CIAT II may produce significant improvement in everyday speech. Further studies comparing CIAT, CIAT II, conventional speech therapy, and no treatment, are planned using a larger subject group."

Review Article: "Intensive Language-Action Therapy (ILAT): The Methods." Friedmann Pulvemuller, MD, Brain Language Laboratory, Department of Philosophy and Humanities, Freie University of Berlin, Berlin, Germany, et. al., Aphasiology, 26: 11, 1317-1351, January, 2013.

Dr. Pulvemuller and his colleagues reviewed many of the recent studies including some in which he was involved. The typical protocol calls for three hours a day for ten to fifteen week-days. Each patient must be assessed to measured deficiencies. Therefore, intervention exercises vary accordingly. Two intervention exercises frequently used are explained below.

(1). Similar intervention exercises that are used in conventional speech therapy are used in CIAT but the difference lies in intensity (3 hours a day) in a short period of time (ten to fifteen days). This could include answering questions in a complete sentence; or looking at a picture of different objects with different colors. The patient is asked to identify the objects and the colors using sentences.

(2). Language Action Games such as the game "Go Fish," are played with a therapist, a volunteer, or even another aphasia patient. Each is given a certain amount of cards with different objects. Each player tries to get matches by asking for a card using a complete sentence.

Conclusions: In the four articles authored by Dr. Pulvemuller, I drew the following conclusions:

(1). There is still a lack of detailed guidance on how to implement practical procedures in clinical settings and how to adjust the method to the variety of deficits of individual patients.

(2). CIAT can improve language performance for patients suffering even from chronic post-stroke aphasia and is considerably more effective than traditional therapy.

(3). Intensity (3 hours per day) and in a short period of time (ten to fifteen week-days) are key to implementing CIAT.

(4). Only trained professionals should implement CIAT.

I asked Dr. Pulvemuller if he believed it will be possible in the future to improve language and speech using CIAT even years post stroke. He answered, "It has proven to work very well already with chronic post stroke aphasia."

Repetitive Transcranial Magnetic Stimulation (rTMS) and Transcranial Direct Current Stimulation (tDCS): These two therapies were discussed at length in chapter one as a rehabilitation treatment for upper limb paralysis after a stroke. They are both also being studied for treatment of aphasia. Both of these therapies have the same goals and the same delivery method. But, where rTMS is delivered by using an electromagnetic coil, tDCS uses two small nine volt batteries. For more information on how these two therapies work, see chapter one. Like Constraint Induced Language Therapy, there are several studies completed or in progress. Below are two such studies and a review.

Study: "Effects of Repetitive Transcranial Magnetic Stimulation in Aphasic Stroke," Thiel, Alexander, MD, PhD et. al., Department of Neurology and Neurosurgery, McGill University at Jewish General Hospital, Montreal, Canada, Stroke, 2011; 42:409-415.

Study concluded 2011

Patients who were in the sub-acute stage of stroke were given multiple sessions of 1 Hz rTMS over the right hemisphere for a two year period. All patients were within sixteen weeks post stroke. In addition, patients received conventional speech and language therapy.

Results: Improvement was significant in all patients receiving rTMS. The researchers concluded that the results of this study should encourage larger clinical trials to explore long-term effectiveness.

Study: "Excitatory rTMS Induces Improvements in Chronic Post-Stroke Aphasia," Jerzy P. Szaflaarski M.D., Donald L. Gilbert, M.D., Jennifer J. Vannest, PhD, et. al., Department of Neurology, University of Cincinnati Children's Hospital, Dept. of Neurology, Medical Science Monitor, 2011; 17(3):132-139.

Study concluded 2011

Eight patients with moderate to severe aphasia as a result of stroke were studied. Each patient was given ten daily treatments of 200 seconds of rTMS to the left hemisphere using an excitatory stimulation method called intermittent theta burst stimulation.

Results: Six of the eight patients showed improved language skills. None of the patients reported ill effects from the treatment. The researchers stated that, "This rTMS protocol appears to be safe and should be further tested in blinded studies assessing its short and long term safety/efficiency for post-stroke aphasia rehabilitation."

Review: In 2013, Dr. Priyanka P. Shah, Dr. Jane Allendorfer, and others wrote a review of the status of non-invasive brain stimulation such as rTMS and tDCS. The review entitled, "Induction of Neuroplasticity and Recovery in Post-Stroke Aphasia by Non-invasive Brain Stimulation," was published in Frontiers in Human Neuroscience in December, 2013. The review stated, "A number of research studies employing these techniques, especially rTMS, have reported lasting improvement in language functions in patients with chronic post-stroke aphasia." The review further states, "Neurorehabilitation of post-stroke aphasia with the use of non-invasive brain stimulation shows a lot of promise."

Drug Therapy for Aphasia: There are several drugs that I found being studied to improve aphasia after a stroke. These include memantine, levetiracetam (Kepra), donepezil, bromocriptine, piracetam, and a group of drugs classified as amphetamines. A summary of results follows.

Memantine: This drug has traditionally been used to treat Alzheimer's disease. A study entitled "Memantine and Constraint Induced Aphasia Therapy in Chronic Post-Stroke Aphasia" concluded in 2009. The principal investigator was Marcelo Berthier MD, PhD. The result was that all twenty seven of the subjects improved with the drug treatment and with CIAT alone but best outcomes were achieved when combining memantine with CIAT. Benefits were maintained after a long-term follow-up evaluation.

Levetiracetam (Kepra): This drug has been traditionally used to treat epilepsy. A 2010 case study gave a traumatic brain injured adult man levetiracetam treatment along with intensive speech therapy. The result was significant improvement in speech and language skills. There is an ongoing study entitled "Levetiracetam to Improve Chronic Aphasia in Post-Stroke Patients." The principal investigator is A.M. Barrett, MD, Kessler Foundation, West Orange, NJ. Fifty stroke patients with aphasia are presently being studied. Each patient receives 250 Mg of Lev orally twice daily for seven days. This is followed by 500 Mg of Lev orally twice daily for seven days. And finally each will receive 1,000 Mg of Lev orally for seven days. This study was not completed at the time of this writing and preliminary results were not available.

Donepezil: This drug has traditionally been used to treat Alzheimer's disease. The most recent study that I found was completed in 2010 entitled "The Efficacy of donepezil for Post-Stroke Aphasia: A Pilot Study." The principal investigator was Y. Chen. Published in Europe PubMed Central, 49_(2)115-118. Sixty patients were given 5 Mg of donepezil daily for twelve weeks. The results showed significant improvement in spontaneous speech, comprehension, repetition, and naming objects.

Bromocriptine: This drug has been used to treat Parkinson 's disease and Type 2 Diabetes. I found several studies, the last of which was in 2000, which showed mixed results using bromocriptine. There are no present studies using bromocriptine in progress.

Piracetam: This drug has been traditionally used to treat myoclonus (involuntary muscle twitching). Like bromocriptine, I found several studies, the last of which was in 2000, which showed mixed results. There are no present studies using piracetam in progress.

Amphetamines: This classification of drugs is used for a variety of disorders including ADHD and narcolepsy. I was able to reach Dr. Delaina Walker-Batson, PhD, Professor and Director of the Stroke Center-Dallas, T. Boone Pickens Institute of Health Services, Texas Woman's College, Dallas, Texas. Dr. Walker-Batson directed me to a 2013 review she wrote entitled "Amphetamine and Post-Stroke Rehabilitation: Indications and Controversies," for the European Journal of Physical and Rehabilitation Medicine, 49:2, 2013, April, pgs. 251-260.

Dr. Walker-Batson states in her review, "While the experimental literature continues to mount for an AMPH effect, the translation to clinical trials has been less clear. This is due in part to the inherent difficulty extrapolating results in animals to humans." Further, "While evidence from the basic science laboratory has continued to increase in support of AMPH facilitation of post-stroke deficits, the results of the limited number of clinical studies are far from clear, and bring up numerous controversies and questions." "Dr. Walker-Batson concludes that as a result of the present studies, it is apparent that both research methods and rehabilitation practices need to be redesigned to use smaller trials to answer specific questions such as:

+ How long post-stroke will yield the best results?
+ How much treatment (dose, length of treatment, etc.) will yield the best results? Only then can larger trials take place to measure the success of amphetamine treatment in treating post-stroke aphasia."

Chapter 4: Alexia: Promising Research

"Our greatest weakness is giving up. The most certain way to succeed is always to try just one more time" Thomas Edison

Alexia is the term used when someone loses the ability to read or understand words, sentences, or, in some cases, even recognize letters. It is also called acquired dyslexia, visual aphasia or word blindness. This is fairly common after a stroke. It is caused by damage to the left side of the brain (usually the occipital and temporal lobes). Alexia and dyslexia are terms that are often used interchangeably. However, developmental dyslexia, a problem with learning how to read and write in the first place, is different from acquired alexia. Alexia is a reading disability acquired as a result of an event such as a stroke. It is quite common for alexia to be accompanied by expressive aphasia (the inability to speak in sentences), and agraphia (the inability to write).

All alexia is not the same, however. A person may have difficulty with: recognizing words, identifying and reading synonyms, reading narrative despite his ability to sound out and pronounce words, reading for very long, blind spots blocking the end of a line or a long word, focusing on the left side of the paragraph or page, double vision when trying to read, not being able to read some words, or any combination of these traits, which makes reading impossible.

Trying to overcome alexia is difficult because:

+ There are several types of alexia, so treatments will be different depending on the type of alexia to be treated.
+ Treatment for a particular type of alexia may help one patient and not another.

So let us look at the different types of alexia. There are two categories; **Peripheral Alexia and Central Alexia.**

Peripheral Alexia: Alexia in this category centers on visual blockage. It includes hemianopic alexia, neglect alexia, and attentional alexia.

Hemianopic Alexia is the most common of the peripheral category. There is visual field loss due to damage to the primary visual cortex. Sometimes this loss can be up to 50% of the visual field. A right- sided hemianopia results in difficulty with normal left-to-right reading as patients cannot see up-coming words.

Neglect Alexia results in a reader having a problem identifying the beginning of a word. For example, the reader might misread the word "stone" as "tone." The reader has neglected the first letter. The reader may see "dog" instead of "log." The reader misread the first letter of the word which made a different word.

Attentional Alexia results in the reader seeing crowded letters sometimes blending two words into one. The lack of spacing between words makes reading slow and difficult. This is most commonly seen in a rare form of dementia called "posterior cortical atrophy."

Central Alexia: Patients who have central alexia have a general language disorder. The alexia is part of expressive aphasia. The reader cannot read very well but also will have problems talking and writing. This category includes phonological alexia, deep alexia, pure alexia, and surface alexia.

Phonological Alexia is a very common form of alexia. It results in the reader being able to read words that they recognize but not words that are unfamiliar to them. Readers with phonological alexia cannot sound out written words easily.

Deep Alexia has all of the features of phonological alexia, but the reader also makes errors with words saying a related meaning instead of the correct meaning. For example, the word to be read is "cat" but the reader reads "dog." The reader reads "fast" instead of "slow." Many researchers characterize deep alexia as a severe version of phonological alexia and treatment options are the same.

<u>Pure Alexia</u> results in the reader being able to recognize and name individual letters but has difficulty reading words. The reader also has difficulty with sequence of words. Many therapists call this letter-by-letter reading because the reader cannot recognize words as a whole object and must assemble them from their parts. Usually the patient can write a sentence normally but then cannot easily read what he/she has written.

<u>Surface Alexia</u> is basically the opposite of phonological alexia. The reader may not have difficulty with words where pronunciations are regular (consistent with their spelling) such as "hand" or "bat" (especially single syllable words). However, the reader will have difficulty with phonologically irregular words such as "colonel" or "patient" or "scent."

Studies and Treatment: At the time of this writing, I could find no studies being done on alexia other than phonological, hemianopic, and pure alexia. I looked at many studies or trials for alexia, all of which were small. More studies are needed.

Phonological Alexia Studies and Treatment:

The studies that I looked at used multi methods, some of which had some success. Almost all of the studies required more trials and the methods used would be difficult or impossible for a patient to use on his own.

The exception is a method called LiPS (Lindamood Phonemy Sequencing Program). Several researchers used LiPS in their studies and found significant improvement in reading speed and spelling.

The LiPS program helps patients to identify the sequence of sounds within words going through a series of steps. This method helps the patient differentiate between words by developing the ability to sound out words. Words unfamiliar to the reader will be more easily identified. Readers are taught to self monitor and correct their own errors during reading and spelling. You can go to the LiPS web-site to get more information.

Hemianoptic Alexia Studies and Treatment:

In every hemianopic alexia study that I have read, the same type of therapy was used and recommended. The therapy is called "Read-Right." Using this method, studies have shown great improvement and even total return to normal reading in some cases.

The therapy entails a written text sliding across a computer screen from right to left. The client controls the speed and selects the content (history, literature, current events, etc.).

Best of all, the program is free and accessible to all on the internet by typing in "Read-Right" in a search engine such as Google. You must then register on the Read Right web-site.

Pure Alexia Studies and Treatment:

I have read several studies for treatment of pure alexia. The best success was using what researchers call "tactile-kinesthetic" treatment to improve a patient's letter recognition and reading speed.

Tactile-kinesthetic means using the sense of touch and movement to recognize letters and later words. The patients were instructed to write each letter of the alphabet on the palms of their left hands with a capped pen. The left hand produced the sense of touch and feeling (tactile), while the right hand produced the sense of movement (kinesthetic).

To increase speed, the patients practiced naming letters, then groups of letters, and finally words. Researchers believe that tactile-kinesthetic techniques train the brain to remember letters by feeling and movement rather than by vision.

Another approach used a technique called "Multiple Oral Reading." MOR focuses on re-reading a given text 30 minutes a day for one week. At the end of each week there was an evaluation of speed and accuracy and a new text was given each week. The study lasted two months. A similar study using the same approach lasted almost a year. These studies resulted in significant reading improvement.

The results of these studies, however, for me, are problematic. All of the pure alexia studies that I found involved either a very small group or in some cases, an individual case study.

How do you combat Alexia? First, have a speech-language pathologist with experience with alexia do a formal diagnosis. He/she will be able to pinpoint the type of alexia that you have and suggest possible treatments and strategies. He/she will also be aware of the latest studies and treatments available. Next, get a low vision examination by an ophthalmologist (not an optometrist) who has experience with alexia. If the problem is primarily damage to the visual field, he might be able to prescribe corrective lenses or be familiar with techniques to improve reading eye movements.

You can also try the following at-home tips and treatments: *

+ Silent reading is easier than reading out loud. The difficulty of word retrieving in speech is also difficult for reading out loud.
+ Sound out individual letters and letter combinations. "s" would be the sssssss sound.
+ Combination sounds would include "th" "sh" "ch" "st" "bl" "ph" "br" etc. This requires many practice sessions between the survivor and an aide. Many words can be read correctly by sounding out

the letters and then blending the sounds to make a word. In other words, once you learn to sound out the first letter or combination, the letters can blend into words.

+ Some survivors are able to pronounce words that are spelled out to them. Start out with simple words such as c-a-r or h-a-t. Then move on to longer words such as a-n-i-m-a-l. Then move on to sentences such as l-o-o-k a-t t-h-e a-n-i-m-a-l.

+ For nouns, try pairing the word with a picture of the object. The aide can then use these words in a sentence without the pictures so that reading takes place.

+ Some survivors cannot read due to visual attention. They can't focus on one word at a time. Try cutting a "window" out of a piece of paper to block out all but one word at a time.

+ Some patients can read words but they get confused as to when the line ends. By putting a solid bookmark at the end of the paragraph, column, or page, these survivors may find that this method reduces confusion and helps in reading concentration. If the problem is finding the beginning of each sentence, put the bookmark at the beginning of each paragraph, column, or page.

+ Some survivors have a blind spot which blocks the end of lines or even the end of a long word. So "backward" may look like "back". Patients can be trained to look at the last letter in long words first and the last word of each sentence first. You can also try turning the text 90 degrees clockwise to read.

+ Other vision related alexia may be able to be corrected by the above mentioned ophthalmologist prescribing glasses.

+ If you can read but with difficulty, try large print books and magazines such as Reader's Digest Large Print. This helped a survivor that I know. You can also enjoy books on CD's which are now available at any book store.

Sources used for Phonological Alexia:

Kendell, Diane; Conway, Timothy; Rosenbek, John; Gonzalez-Rothi, Leslie (2003). "Case Study

Phonological Rehabilitation of Acquired Phonologic Alexia." Aphasiology 17(11): 1073-1095.

Beeson, PM; Rising, K; Kim, ES; Rapcsak, SZ (April, 2010). "A Treatment Sequence for Phonological Alexia/Agraphia." J. Speech Lang Hear Res 53 (2): 450-468.

The LiPS (Lindamood Phonemy Sequencing Program) web-site.

Lindamood, P. & Lindamood, P. (1998). "The Lindamood Phonemy Sequencing Program for Reading, Spelling, and Speech." (Teachers Manual in the Classroom and Clinic). Austin, Texas: Pro-Ed.

Sperling, AJ; Lott, SN; Snider, S; Ferguson, S; Friedman, RB. "A New Treatment For Phonological Text Alexia." Brain and Language 95 (2005) 209-210.

Beeson, PM, & Insalaco, D. (1998). "Acquired Alexia: Lesson From Successful Treatment." Journal of International Neuropsychological Society, 4: 621-635.

Leff, AP, & Schofield, T. "Rehabilitation of Acquired Alexia." In: JH Stone, M Blouin, editors. International Encyclpedia of Rehabilitation.

Conway, Timothy, & Kendell, Diane. (Oct., 2013). "Multimodal Treatment of Phonological Alexia: Behavioral & fMRI Outcomes." The Aphasiology Archive: University of Pittsburgh.

Sources Used for Hemianopic Alexia:
Leff, Alexander P.; Ong, Y.H.; Brown, MM; Robinson, P.; Plant, G.T.; Husain, M.; (2012). "Read-Right: a "Web App" That Improves Reading Speeds in Patients with Hemianopia." Journal of Neurology. (12): 2611-2615.

Schuett, S. (2009), "The Rehabilitation of Hemianopic Dyslexia." National Review Neurology. (8): 427-437.

Spitzyna G.A.; Wise R.J.S.; McDonald S.A.; Plant G.T.; Kidd D.; Crewes H.; Leff A.P. "Optokinetic Therapy Improves Text Reading in Patients With Hemianopic Alexia." Neurology. May 29, 2007: 68 (22) 1922-1930.

Sources Used for Pure Alexia:
Susan Nitzburg Lott, Aimee Syms Carney, and Rhonda B. Friedman. "Overt Use of a Tactile-Kinesthetic Strategy Shifts to Convert Processing in Rehabilitation of Letter-By-Letter Reading." Aphasia November, 2010: 24 (11) 1424-1442.

Susan Nitzburg Lott and Rhonda B. Friedman. 1999: "Can Treatment for Pure Alexia Improve Letter-By-Letter Reading Speed Without Sacrificing
Accuracy." Brain and Language 67, 188-201.

Moyer SB. "Rehabilitation of Acquired Alexia." Cortex 15, (1979): 139-142.

Pelagie Beeson, Joel Magloire, and Randall Robey. "Letter-By-Letter Reading: Natural Recovery and Response to Treatment." Behavioral Neurology 16 (2005) 191-202.

---

* Much of the information on at-home treatments came from the article "Reading Rehab", by Margaret Greenwald PhD, STROKE CONNECTION MAGAZINE, July/August, 2004

Part II: Problems and Solutions for Stroke Survivors

Chapter 5: Dealing With the Five Disabilities after a Stroke

"The goal of stroke rehabilitation is to restore as much independence as possible by improving physical, mental, and emotional functions"
<u>Hope: The Stroke Recovery Guide</u>

The degree of motor damage and cognitive damage as a result of a stroke varies greatly from patient to patient because of the part of the brain affected or damaged and how badly the brain was damaged. In this article, I have examined the five categories of disabilities and how a survivor can deal with each.

1. **Movement dysfunction and paralysis:** If a stroke happens on the left side of the brain, it will affect the right side of the body. A right brain stroke will affect the left side of the body.

a. Paralysis can be on either side of the body. It can be of the foot and leg, the arm and hand, or both. If there is total paralysis, there is no treatment to improve or reverse that condition.

b. Dysphagia, or difficulty swallowing, occurs in some patients but is usually greatly reduced or cured early on by a speech therapist.

c. Ataxia affects the body's ability to coordinate movement which leads to difficulties with body posture, balance, and walking.

d. Spasticity or tone "is a condition where muscles are stiff and resist being stretched. It can be found throughout the body but may be most common in the arms, fingers or legs. Depending on where it occurs, it can result in an arm being pressed against the chest, a stiff knee or a pointed foot that interferes with walking. It can also be accompanied by painful spasms." (Stroke: A Stroke

Recovery Guide, a publication of the National Stroke Association, p. 52).

Treatment Options for partial paralysis, ataxia, and spasticity:

A combination of physical therapy, occupational therapy, and medication is standard treatment.

Exercises for strength, balance, coordination, stretching, or range of motion can be helpful.

A brace on the affected leg to provide support and to correct foot drop is often prescribed.

Injection of Botox into the affected area to relax the muscles by blocking the nerve activity that creates the stiffness has proven to be helpful in some patients.

Baclofen Therapy has been successful for some patients in treating severe spasticity. Baclofen is injected into the spinal fluid using a surgically placed pump, or is sometimes taken orally.

Constraint Induced Movement Therapy has been under experiment and has shown great promise.

It is designed for patients who have arm weakness and spasticity, but the patient must have some ability to move the hand. If you are interested in this research, Google: CIMT Edward Taub.

Research is in progress using stem cells and transcranial magnetic stimulation with the goal of reversing at least some of the physical damage done by stroke.

2. Sensory dysfunction: In some stroke patients, pathways for sensation are damaged resulting in pain in the side or the limb being blocked. Decreased feeling in the limbs, numbness or burning in the limbs, and pain are examples of sensory dysfunction.

Decreased feeling, usually in the limbs, can occur but is not common.

Tingling, numbness, or burning, usually in the limbs, can occur but is not common.

Pain is the most troubling sensory problem because it is more frequent than the other sensory problems and it is usually more debilitating.

Pain is often caused by nerve damage or sometimes from lack of movement.

Treatment options for sensory dysfunction:

Decreased feeling, tingling, and burning in the limbs is very difficult to treat especially because what works for one patient may not work for another. Some patients report that continuous light exercise brings relief. Acupuncture, heat application, meditation, and prescribed medications are also reported by some to give relief.

Pain is also difficult to treat because pain after a stroke can occur in various parts of the body. I wrote an article in the July, 2013 issue of the strokenetwork.org newsletter where I give tips on reducing pain. These tips are listed below.

Yoga and meditation can help relax and teach the patient to breathe properly.

Progressive Muscle Relaxation (PMR) is a step-by-step technique that helps the patient become aware of muscle tension and reduces the tension through a systematic approach that reduces pain. You can look at the PMR web-site to see visuals that will walk you through the PMR exercises.

The Trigger Point Therapy Workbook: Your Treatment Guide For Pain Relief by Clare Davies has received good reviews on Amazon. Readers should give this therapy a try.

Chronic pain deserves treatment by a pain management specialist, and/or acupuncturist.

3. Problems with language: Language difficulties include the ability to speak, understand, write, read, add and subtract. All of these problems occur as a result of a left brain stroke.

Aphasia, which has many components, can be simplified by using just two terms. Expressive aphasia is the lack of ability to verbally express thoughts or to write sentences. The survivor can understand what is said, but can respond with only one word or just a few words. Sometimes speech can be extremely slow, while other patients speak so rapidly it is difficult to understand them. The second category is receptive aphasia. Sounds are heard but the patient cannot understand what was said or written. (Chapter 3 deals with aphasia and promising research).

Alexia means the lack of the ability to read. My experience is that both expressive and receptive aphasia patients experience difficulty in reading. (Chapter 4 deals with alexia and ongoing research).

Agraphia simply means the lack of ability to write. This usually, but not always, goes along with Alexia.

Acalculia is the loss of mathematical ability including addition, subtraction, division, and multiplication.

Treatment options for problems with language:

There is no treatment for agraphia or for acalculia. However, successful treatment for alexia may also improve agraphia and acalculia. For treatment options for aphasia, see chapter 3. For treatment options for alexia, see chapter 4.

4. Problems with Memory and Reasoning: Stroke can result in problems with short term memory, judgment, and also the ability to plan, comprehend meaning, learn new tasks, and solve problems.

Apraxia is the impairment or loss of ability to carry out learned movements despite having the desire and the physical ability to perform the movements.

Anosognosia is a deficit of awareness. The patient seems unaware of the existence of his or her disability.

Treatment options for problems with memory and reasoning:

Most stroke survivors recognize their short term memory loss and are able to adjust to it. Cognitive therapists develop strategies such as keeping a daily planner which focuses on organizing activities one day at a time.

There is little consensus on assessing apraxia but treatment includes speech, occupational and physical therapy. Some patients show significant improvement while others do not. Unfortunately, those patients that do not respond to therapy may not be able to function independently. There is no drug available to treat apraxia.

No long term treatment is known to help anosognosia, however, the condition usually disappears in time.

5. Problems with Emotion: Many people experience a range of emotional changes after a stroke. These changes can cause the person's personality to change and can be disruptive and problematic.

Depression is a common condition after a stroke. It can be mild or it can be all consuming. Although depression is a normal part of grief after a stroke, if it continues for the long run, professional help is called for.

Anger is also common after a stroke. In my support group, once every two months we split into two groups; one for survivors and one for caregivers. Many times I have heard a caregiver complain about fits of anger from their loved one for no apparent reason.

Emotional Lability is a condition of the brain that causes sudden, uncontrollable crying or inappropriate laughter. Of course this can result in embarrassing situations for both the survivor and the caregiver.

Apathy is not the same as depression even though the behavior is similar. The survivor who is apathetic cannot seem to get motivated. He stays in bed too long, sits or lies on the couch for hours, and often will not leave the house.

Anxiety is an unpleasant feeling which often includes nervous behavior such as wringing the hands or pacing about. It is a feeling of fear or distress over something that is unlikely to occur such as a heart attack or car accident.

Treatment options for problems with emotion:

Antidepressants, drugs that control mood, psychological counseling, and psychiatric therapy are treatments for depression, anxiety, and anger management.

Apathy is more difficult to treat because there are no drugs available to treat it. However, therapists and counselors have had success by developing a routine for the patient to follow. This includes getting up every day at the same time and scheduling events or activities at certain times each day. The focus is on action which will later lead to motivation toward everyday life.

I could not find any treatment for emotional lability, but fortunately after a few months, it usually (but not always) fades away.

I wrote an article in the September, 2012 issue of strokenetwork.org on anger and aggressive behavior. There are drugs that are sometimes successful in treating this problem, but there is much the caregiver can do to lessen anger.

+ Remember that anger and aggressive behavior are a result of the stroke. Your loved one cannot always control this behavior.
+ Stay calm. Do not overreact to your loved one's outbursts. Speak slowly and softly without raising your voice until your loved one calms down.
+ Avoid arguing or confrontation with your loved one. Redirect her attention to something else.
+ After you identify things that create anger in your loved one, avoid them as much as

possible. For example, if you observe that being around a large group of people sets him/her off, avoid that environment.

+   If you as a caregiver become angry or frustrated, back off and cool down. Chances are he/she will also calm down after you step back and remain calm.

+   Stay safe. If your loved one becomes violent, back away keeping a safe distance, and seek help if need be.

Chapter 6: Seizures after a Stroke

"From the brain and from the brain only, arise our pleasures, joys, laughters, and jests, as well as our sorrows, grief, and tears" Hippocrates

Many people without stroke knowledge mistake a seizure for a stroke because they can look the same as they occur. Strokes and Seizures should not be confused. They are vastly different. A seizure is usually brief and the person recovers after a short time. A stroke is a longer episode and almost always leaves some kind of permanent damage.

Joan Lippert, Managing Editor of Publications at Albert Einstein College of Medicine, explains the difference between stroke and seizure. "A seizure happens when a brief, strong surge of electrical activity affects part or all of the brain. Nerve cells in your brain conduct the electricity.

Cells that are chemically or physically unstable may become too active, conduct too much electricity, and activate nearby nerves. A stroke interferes with the brain's blood supply. When a blood vessel that carries oxygen and nutrients to the brain is either blocked by a clot (ischemic) or bursts (hemorrhagic) a stroke will occur. In both types of stroke, the surrounding area of the brain can't get the blood and oxygen it needs, and it starts to die within two to three minutes." ("Stroke and Seizure," Joan Lippert, Heart Insight, May, 2008).

But what causes a stroke survivor to experience seizures more commonly than people who have not had a stroke? First some facts.

1. Between 10% and 22% of stroke survivors experience seizures until several years post stroke. (In one article that I read, the authors put the figure at 10%. However, the Epilepsy Foundation puts the number at 22%.)

2. In the elderly, just over half of newly diagnosed cases of epilepsy are related to a previous stroke. The Stroke Registry reports that of the approximate 500,000 to 700,000

people who experience strokes each year, about 36,500 will have seizures post stroke.

3. Seizures post stroke are slightly more apt to happen in cases of hemorrhagic rather than ischemic stroke.

4. Seizure risk after a stroke is greatest within the first thirty days post stroke.

5. Seizures become a greater risk after a second stroke.

According to Ralph L. Sacco, M.D., professor of neurology and epidemiology at Columbia University Medical Center, "Seizures occur whenever there is a scar on the brain. When stroke injures part of the brain, it leaves a scar, and this scar can then trigger abnormal electrical activity that can start a seizure." ("Controlling Post-Stroke Seizures," Mike Mills, Stroke Connection Magazine, January/February, 2006).

Types of Seizures as published in Neurology Now, Aug./Sept., 2013, p. 45.

Absence: brief episode of staring; awareness and responsiveness are impaired

Atypical Absence: periods of staring; individual is somewhat responsive

Myoclonic: brief, shock-like jerks of muscle or group of muscles

Atonic: muscles suddenly lose strength; eyelids may droop; head may nod; person may fall to the ground

Tonic: muscle tone greatly increased; stiffening of arms, legs common; person usually remains conscious

Clonic: rhythmic jerking movements of the arms and/or legs; confusion after seizure

Tonic-clonic: also known as *grand mal*; loss of consciousness; involves the entire body; this type of seizure is what most people think of when they hear the word "seizure"

If you see someone having a seizure:

1. Roll the person on one side to prevent choking on fluids or vomit.
2. Cushion the person's head.
3. Loosen any tight clothing around the neck.
4. Keep the person's airway open. If need be, tilt the person's head back.

5. Never put anything in the person's mouth (especially your hand or fingers).
6. Do not restrict the person from moving unless in danger.
7. Remove any sharp or solid objects that the person might hit during the seizure.
8. Note how long the seizure lasts and what symptoms occurred. You can then inform emergency medical personnel.
9. Stay with the person until the seizure ends or until emergency personnel arrive.

Information from <u>Stroke Connection Magazine,</u> Jan. /Feb., 2006. p.16.

Treating seizures after a stroke:
Although doctors have a good understanding of what causes seizures and how to treat seizures, there is no cure. They do know that treating seizures at early onset, usually with specific medications, will result in decreased risk for recurring seizures. However, there is still risk for long term seizures.

Treating seizures post stroke is the same as treating epilepsy. That is, the same drugs are given for both epileptic and post stroke seizures. There are presently

54 anti seizure drugs approved either by the FDA (Food and Drug Administration) or by similar regulators in other countries. These medications can be divided into "narrow-spectrum anti-seizure medications," designed to treat specific types of seizures, and "broad-spectrum anti-seizure medications," designed to treat a wide variety of seizures types.

When doctors prescribe an appropriate medication for a patient, they will consider side effects to be avoided, convenience of use, cost, insurance coverage, and type of seizure diagnosed.

Narrow-spectrum	Broad-spectrum
(Brand names)	(Brand names)
Dilantin	Depakote
Sabril	Lamictal
Tegretol	Topamax
Trileptal	Zonagran
Neurontin	Keppra
Lyrica	Klonopin
Vimpat	Banzel

(some medications containing phenobarbital may also be prescribed)

Every seizure medication can have side effects. These may include fatigue, dizziness, unsteadiness, blurry vision, stomach upset, headaches, reduced resistance from colds, and memory loss. This is just a partial list and these side effects are usually temporary. There are, however, some rare but serious side effects that can occur. These include problems with blood count, depression with suicidal thoughts, and possible liver damage. Each individual drug will come with a package insert to list that drug's possible side effects. It is important for patients taking an anti-seizure drug to read that insert carefully.

Chapter 7: I Want to Return to Work

"A well spent day brings happy sleep" Leonardo DaVinci

Some stroke survivors are able to go back to work within a short time after their stroke or traumatic brain injury (TBI), even at the same job they had held before. Some can go back to work after an extended recovery. Some can go back to work to a different job, perhaps only part-time. And some can never return to work. The important thing for stroke and TBI survivors, however, is to accept what will be best for them to accomplish their goals.

Going back to work can be therapeutic. It can be challenging. It can be rewarding. But it can also be frustrating. The survivor must overcome both physical and cognitive challenges.

When to go back to work: In the support group that I attend, I have heard many brain injury survivors speak about how they went back to work too soon. It was suggested that there are three people to consult when making the decision about going back to work. First, listen to what your loved one and caregiver think. Second, ask your doctor, ideally your neurologist, if he thinks you are able to work. The doctor can help you plan, not only when to go back to work, but also how many hours that you can handle and the type of job where you can be successful. And third, you are most important in determining your own abilities, desires, motivation, and stamina.

Going back to your old job: Will you need special accommodations if you return to your previous job? Will you be able to function in the same position you had held, or will you need to be placed in a position where there is less responsibility? Will you need to work fewer hours than you did before your stroke? And, how much do you want to reveal about your brain injury to your employer and co-workers? If you will need special accommodations, obviously you will have to discuss this with your supervisor. You must get an honest feeling about how enthusiastic your employer is about having you return to the job and if he is willing to offer accommodations to help you succeed.

Working without losing your benefits: In the support group, I frequently hear from survivors who want to try going back to work but are afraid of losing their Social Security benefits and Medicare and/or Medicaid benefits. It is important to find out if other benefits, such as housing assistance, assistance with medications, veteran benefits, etc. will be affected if you begin working.

If you do want to explore working, you should start by visiting the local office of your state division of vocational rehabilitation. I believe every state (also Canada) has such an office or its equivalent. They will offer valuable help with vocational testing, training, and job counseling. They will also explain the Ticket to Work Program.

Ticket to Work Program: The Ticket to Work Program is for people who are receiving SSDI or SSI benefits from Social Security and want to explore working without losing Social Security, Medicare, and Medicaid benefits. You must select an Employment Network (EN) so that you can obtain employment services or other support services. The EN will verify your eligibility by contacting the Operations Manager. Your vocational rehabilitation office will be an EN and may also be able to give you names and locations of other EN's in your area. EN's are agencies that have an agreement with the Social Security Administration to provide the above mentioned services to eligible recipients. You may visit several EN locations to see which one is best for you before accepting their ticket to work services.

Part of the Ticket to Work Program includes "Work Incentives," which allow you to keep your Medicaid and Medicare benefits and your SSDI or SSI benefits in full during a nine month trial work period, regardless of how much you earn, provided you report your work and income to Social Security. The nine months do not have to be consecutive but rather any nine months out of the next 60 months. Also, any month where you do not earn a "Substantial Gainful Activity"

(SGA) the amount will not count towards the nine months of trial work. After this Trial Work period, if you continue to earn below the SGA minimum, you will not lose SSI or SSDI benefits. The amount you can earn under SGA depends on your geographic location and other factors. Your Vocational Rehabilitation office can advise you on this. Any Social Security office will have booklets explain "Ticket to Work" and "Employment after a Disability."

I hope this article takes some of the fear out of trying to go back to work. If you are uncertain, try volunteering first to help you determine your stamina and your physical and cognitive abilities. Remember to get input from your family and your doctor, and, above all from the counselors at the Vocational Rehabilitation office near you.

Chapter 8: Multi Tasking after a Stroke

"If the brain were simple enough to understand it, we would be too simple to understand it" Peter Bognanni (novelist)

I do not have to define multi tasking because it is obvious in our daily lives. When we drive a car, we must be cognizant of the speed we are going, traffic on the road, signs to tell us where to get off the highway, remembering to use the turn signal, changing lanes, all while listening to the radio. Think of the things you do on the job that require multi tasking: dealing with budgets, dealing with fellow workers, dealing with the problems you must fix, and dealing with deadlines, all while listening to the radio.

If you are a parent, you must multi task every day. The kids must be off to school. Shopping must be organized. You must get to work on time. And that is just in the morning. You have other things to do in the afternoon and evening.

But after one has a stroke, especially a right brain stroke, multi tasking can be extremely difficult. The survivor must focus on a two part solution. First, try to limit or reduce multi tasking where possible. Second, practice techniques designed to improve multi tasking after a stroke.

Reducing Multi Tasking:
A former corporate executive stroke survivor has trained himself to complete one single task before moving on to the next task. Others I have read about say removing distractions is a way of maximizing concentration so the survivor can totally focus on the task at hand. I have read about many other survivors who have encountered typical problems and offer how they deal with them. When out walking with a friend, one survivor said she has to block out other people walking to be able to focus on the conversation with her friend.

One man says he always turns the radio off while driving and often verbally reminds himself to keep the right speed and to be aware of other drivers on the road. A woman survivor states that she cannot listen to music and listen to someone talking to her at the same time.

I mentor a woman that suffered a stroke fourteen years ago. She has several disabilities including expressive aphasia and right-side paralysis. Whenever I talk to her about a new medication or a problem she is having, I make her turn off the TV. If she does not, she will not understand my directions. When I am talking to her, I cannot give her more than one thought or she may forget both. An example of this took place recently. I called her to remind her that I would be picking her up for a dental appointment the next morning. I also told her that her medication was ready and she should pick it up at this time. When I arrived the next morning, she had forgotten that I was coming and forgot to pick up her medication. You might suspect this was a short term memory problem, but it was not. Whenever I give her just one direction, she never forgets.

Improving Multi Tasking:

In this section, I have described what several survivors have told me about what their cognitive rehabilitation therapists have done or are doing to improve multi tasking.

More than a few survivors have told me that doing jigsaw puzzles, crossword puzzles, and Sudoku number puzzles have been recommended. By starting out with easy puzzles and gradually progressing to more difficult ones, the patient will start thinking about more than one thing at a time. Using a jigsaw puzzle as an example, the patient must not only look at how each piece fits with other pieces, but also how each piece relates to other pieces as part of the picture.

I recently read about a study published in the American Journal of Occupational Therapy about using a "virtual supermarket," to improve multi tasking skills. Each patient was given the task of buying six items from a virtual mall put up on a computer screen, and was asked to find four pieces of information. After four participants practiced this skill in ten 60 minute sessions over a three week period, improvement ranged from 21% to about 52%. This study was very small, however, so conclusions should be viewed with caution.

Another survivor said she plays the match game with cards. A set number of pairs of cards are used with various pictures on them. After shuffling the cards and then laying them face down in rows, each participant takes turns turning over two cards. If you find a match, you take the cards and go again. This goes on until all the pairs are complete. The player with the most cards wins. The more card pairs used, the more difficult the game becomes.

The University of Alabama Birmingham has developed the UAB Home-Based Cognitive Stimulation Program which provides many activities for people post stroke or traumatic brain injury. The activities are done at home on a computer and are designed to improve cognitive skills. There are 48 skills, each with three levels of difficulty. Interested people can go to a search engine such as Google, type in Alabama Birmingham Cognitive Stimulation, and then click on home-based cognitive stimulation activities. This sight also allows you the print out their entire booklet free.

Many of the brain injury survivors in my support group use the web-site Lumosity. It does have a fee but it has a multitude of exercises to improve cognition. It is worth checking out.

Conclusion:

If you find that multi tasking after your stroke or TBI has become difficult, it is advised that you try to limit multi tasking from your daily life. But since it is usually impossible to avoid this completely, try some of the activities listed in this chapter. I must confess that I could not find a single study that definitively concluded that any type of cognitive therapy improved multi tasking. That said, many of the survivors that I questioned felt that the various techniques that I listed have improved their multi tasking ability significantly.

The following sources were used to write this chapter:

University of Alabama Birmingham School of Medicine: Traumatic Brain Injury Model System

Information Network,: <u>UAB-TBIMS Home Based Cognitive Stimulation Activities Booklet,</u> Tom Novak, PhD, Jacqueline Blankenship, MCD, 2002.

Livestock.com, "Multitasking Activities for Brain Injury Rehabilitation," Susan Rush, July 16, 2010.

Examiner.com, "Regaining the Ability to Multitask After it is Lost to a Stroke," Sharon Wagoner, June 10, 2010.

Rebecca Dutton blog, "Home After a Stroke: The Only Magic Bullet I've Found," Rebecca Dutton, October 14, 2012.

Chapter 9: Apathy after a Stroke

"Your brain is like a plant. If you plant a seed in it, it will grow into a big idea" Jane King (West Indian poet)

Apathy is the lack of motivation or enthusiasm. When working toward recovery, enjoying activities, or enjoying life in general, if the survivor shows little emotion or feeling, it is a sign of apathy. This differs from depression which is also common in stroke patients. Depression is treated just as it would be in clinical depression. Doctors use medications, therapy sessions, and in extreme cases, electroconvulsive therapy or transcranial magnetic stimulation.

Treating apathy is different. The caregiver must realize the apathy is a result of the stroke, and should proceed to get help for the patient. It creates stress for the caregiver, but understand that your loved one is not lazy or uncaring. The family physician and cognitive therapist should be consulted to see if therapy by a neuropsychologist is recommended. Often, medications are prescribed.

Common emotional changes after a stroke: *
> Rapid mood changes
> Excessive crying or laughing for no apparent reason
> Feelings of sadness
> Feelings of hopelessness
> Irritability
> Changes in eating, sleeping, and thinking
> Frustration
> Anxiety
> Anger
> **Apathy**
> Depression

Although this article is about apathy, I list all emotional changes so you the caregiver can easily identify which of these emotions have affected your loved one. Many of these emotions may overlap with apathy.

(* "Let's Talk About Stroke." A publication booklet by the American Heart Association, 2012).

One suggested solution is to establish realistic goals with your loved one. It is a great tool to motivate patients and change behavior. **Difficult goals** are more motivating but I have found that mixing difficult goals with **challenging goals** and **attainable goals** is the right formula. I have used this method with all of the brain injured survivors that I have mentored over the last fourteen years. Difficult goals are a challenge and survivors are likely to strive to achieve them. A difficult goal might be learning to drive again, finding a job, or walking without a brace. Challenging goals require work, but with proper motivation and hard work, the patient has a reasonably good chance of reaching such goals. Goals in this category that I have used include quitting smoking, walking faster without a cane, etc. Attainable goals assure success and can accomplish something that is important to the patient such as joining a support group or attending church.

Another suggested solution for the caregiver is to try various methods to motivate the survivor in his daily life such as:

a. Find interesting tasks that your loved one can do without help such as writing long overdue letters or reading a book, etc.

b. Keep to a daily routine such as getting up and going to bed at the same time each day and eating, exercising, taking a shower or bath, and watching a favorite TV show at the same time each day.

c. Ask family and friends to visit as often as they can. Perhaps some can have the occasional lunch or dinner with your loved one.

d. Shower your loved one with praise. Make activities fun and use humor in your conversation.

Helping your loved one cope with apathy:

a. Try to stay calm and relaxed. Remember, apathy is part of the illness.

b. Attend a support group with your loved one. Many positive things come out of a support group. Hearing caregivers with similar problems, meeting stroke survivors with similar problems, attending social events through the support group are just a few benefits.

c. Be sure you and your loved one both get enough exercise.

d. Be sure your loved one gets enough rest. Fatigue is common so a mid-day nap might be advisable.

e. Point out the progress your loved one has achieved. Celebrate both the big and small gains.

Conclusion:

Apathy, along with other emotional problems may occur after a stroke. Apathy is part of stroke symptoms and is not due to laziness. Take action to help your loved one to overcome apathy by involving professionals and by getting your loved one on a schedule and introducing activities and interests.

Chapter 10: Adult Day Care Center

"A man who dares to waste one hour of time has not discovered the value of life" (Charles Darwin)

Adult day care centers are popping up all over America. They are non- residential facilities that operate every weekday for up to twelve hours per day. Most are professionally staffed and provide daily living needs such as meals, supervised activities, social support, and general supervision.

It is important for the caregiver to visit close-by centers to see what they offer. Caregivers should consider cleanliness, food quality, activities, cost per day, and how their stroke survivor loved ones would fit into that environment.

The goal here is to provide the survivor with socialization, stimulation, and to prevent or delay institutionalization. There are generally two types of adult day care centers. The first type is called "adult social day care," which provides activities, meals, recreation, and some health care, such as making sure the patient takes their medications. The second type is called "adult day health care," which includes activities and recreation, but focuses on more needed health care and various types of therapy. Patients that go to such a center usually have severe medical problems and are at risk of requiring a nursing home.

MetLife (insurance) conducted a national study of adult day care centers in 2010. The findings were published in a booklet produced by MetLife available at metlife.com. The findings include the following:

More than 5,000 adult day care centers are operating in the United States providing care for more than 260,000 older Americans each day.

71% of the centers operate as non-profit facilities and 16% are affiliated with the public sector, usually the county in which they operate.

Daily fees are almost always less than home nursing care and about half the cost of a residential facility. In 2010, the average daily fee for this service nationwide was $62.

On average, there is one direct caregiver for every six participants. Nearly 80% of adult day centers have a nurse on staff.

Nearly 50% of centers have a social worker on staff and about 60% offer case management services.

Although having loved ones participate in an adult day care center may not appeal to them, it is an opportunity for filling a void in their lives and has the added benefit of giving the caregiver freedom to work, or just enjoy the daily freedom. It is up to the participants to determine how many hours they spend each day at the center.

The following is an example of a stroke survivor that I know who presently goes to an adult day care center five days per week. Before attending the center Robert (not his real name), age 64, spent much of his time under the supervision of his wife Jane (not her real name). He was bored and cranky watching television and napping most of the time. His disability includes mild expressive aphasia, weakness of the right arm and leg, and significant cognitive limitations. At our support group, Jane heard a member of the group talking about an adult day care center that her brother attends. After carefully looking into this idea, she enrolled Robert into a day facility five miles from their home. Robert is home all day on weekends.

Jane says the difference in Robert is remarkable. He looks forward to going to his center every day. He likes the food and the activities. Jane now has a part-time job which pays for Robert's day care center fee.

Now for the difficult question. How do you pay for adult day care? Costs vary greatly based on what they offer, size of the facility, and where you live in the country. While an adult day care center is almost never covered by private insurance and is not covered by Medicare, some financial assistance may be available through a federal or state program such as Medicaid, the Older

Americans Act, or programs through the Veterans Administration. You should also check to see if your county of residence may be able to help. In some cases, the caregivers, being freed up of time, could go back to work to earn what it would cost to provide day care for their loved ones.

A second problem is transportation to the facility. Check with the facility, your town, and your county to see what transportation options are available.

Check List for Caregivers: The following is a list for you to ask when you visit an adult day care center. Choose only the items you care about and ask, "Do you offer...."

Counseling	Medication management
Education	Physical therapy
Evening care	Recreational activities
Field trips	Respite care
Health screening	Socialization
Meals	Supervision
Medical care	Transportation to and from the center

Remember, you must shop around for what best suits your needs.

Much of this article came from information from the following two sources:

"Eldercare Locator," Department of Human Services, April, 2012.

"Adult Day Care Services," MetLife.com, 2010.

Chapter 11: A Checklist for Caregivers Before Your Loved One is Discharged from In-Patient Care

"The purpose of our lives is to be happy" The *Dalai Lama*

After a patient finishes rehabilitation and is ready for discharge to come home, it is usually up to a caregiver to cover all bases when it comes to the care of the patient. Over the years I have heard from caregivers concerning problems they had when their loved one was discharged from the hospital, usually because they did not have direction for preparation. I hope this chapter, which has a list of sixteen suggestions, will help future caregivers.

1. Find out what your insurance will cover. Whether you have Medicaid, Medicare, or private insurance, you must find out if it covers out-patient therapy, home care

services, if needed, medications and aids such as a wheelchair, cane, braces, etc.

2. Make sure that you have set up an out-patient therapy schedule for speech, physical, and occupational therapy.

3. Be sure you have prescriptions for needed medications. Be sure you have an understanding of possible side effects and drug interaction.

4. Ask therapists how you can help the patient in assisting them with personal care, at-home physical therapy, wheelchair transfer, etc. Find out if you need any special training for any of the above.

5. Find out if the patient needs to be on a special diet or will he have restrictions on certain foods and drinks.

6. Keep an index card on your refrigerator with important phone numbers. Get these phone numbers before discharge.

7. In case of emergency, know who you should contact. Know who will

accompany the patient to the hospital, and if there are children living in the home, be sure to have a plan for watching them if you must quickly get to the hospital.

8. Make sure you have contacted the patient's school or work place to inform them of the stroke and prognosis for returning to school or the job.

9. Organize a group of folders with all pertinent information including medical records. Always have these ready for phone calls and doctors appointments.

10. Find out if it is safe to leave the patient alone

11. Find out if the therapists recommend special equipment for the home, especially for the shower and bathroom.

12. Be sure to explore all financial resources including Social Security Disability, Medicare, Medicaid, and church funds.

13. Be sure that you have enough comfortable clothing for the patient. This includes shoes that are able to fit over a brace, possibly with Velcro fasteners instead of laces.

14. Find out what transportation resources are available in your area. If the patient is in a wheelchair, eliminate those that do not offer a wheelchair method of entry.

15. Find out what state, county, and community resources are available. The hospital should have a list of these, but the front of a phone book can be helpful in finding other resources.

16. Ask family friends, neighbors, and clergy if they are willing to help with support, visitations, and especially taking over while you take a break, even if the break is just for a few hours each week. Do not wait for them to offer. You should take the initiative.

Chapter 12: Aquatic Therapy After a Stroke

"In each of us there is another whom we do not know" Carl Jung

What is Aquatic Therapy?
Aquatic therapy (also called water therapy, hydrotherapy, and pool therapy) is using a warm water pool facility to perform physical therapy. It is designed to help the survivor using both the buoyancy of the water and the resistance of the water to improve balance, strength, and to reduce chronic pain. It has the additional benefit of reducing or eliminating the fear of falling during the therapy. Warm water therapy offers a safe and relaxing setting to improve physical skills.

Why Aquatic Therapy?
I had never heard of aquatic therapy until I visited the "Y" in Randolph, New Jersey, where I

saw a demonstration using a special treadmill in the therapy pool adjusted so that the water came up to the patient's chest. I was told the water temperature was kept between 85 and 90 degrees.

Until recently, physical therapy applied to stroke survivors was only performed at a gym, in a physical therapy facility, or a rehabilitation hospital. Aquatic therapy in a pool is a wonderful addition to these facilities to perform a different set of physical therapy exercises and movements.

Aquatic therapy gives the patient greater mobility because body weight is decreased significantly (up to 90%) and water buoyancy creates balance making movement easier. Since the water aids balance, the patient has an easier time with flexibility and stretching muscles. Because of the buoyancy that the pool water provides, the patient can stand up with far less physical strength. Some survivors, who cannot walk on land, find they are able to stand up and even walk in a pool.

Aquatic therapy results in strength improvement because the water provides resistance similar to the concept of isometrics. Resistance increases the survivor's ability to regain muscle performance, motor skills, and flexibility.

Aquatic therapy has also been successful in reducing chronic pain. In a warm pool, spasticity (or tone) is reduced during exercise which is often the cause of upper and lower extremity pain. Even head pain may be reduced because the warm water calms the body releasing endorphins, which are natural pain killers. (Much of the information for this section on "Why Aquatic Therapy?" came from: "The Healing Benefits of Water," Lisa Nagg, Stroke Smart Magazine, Winter, 2012.)

Specific Techniques:
Aquatic therapy is often divided into two types: deep water exercises and shallow water exercises.

Deep water exercises use water buoyancy to balance the body in an upright position so that the patient can stretch, walk (sometimes on a treadmill when available), run in place, and perform bicycle movements while holding on to the side of the pool. All of these exercises are much easier in water than in the traditional physical therapy setting.

Shallow water exercises are designed to help the stroke survivor gain strength and balance as a transition to walking on land. Walking in shallow water is the primary exercise. The patient walks around in the pool avoiding obstacles placed randomly on the pool floor. Because the water is no more than knee deep, balance is more difficult, but once that skill is mastered, the patient can transition to land exercises. (Most of the information in "Specific Techniques" above came from "Pool Therapy as Stroke Rehab," Linda Huey, Word Press published on-line, May 3, 2012).

Studies Involving Aquatic Therapy:

In a published case study involving a stroke patient who received aquatic therapy at Vital Energy Wellness and Rehab Center in Lexington, South Carolina, the results were as follows: The patient suffered right side paralysis resulting from a stroke and was unable to stand, walk or perform other normal functions. After aquatic therapy, she experienced decreased pain and had improved muscle strength and balance. She is now able to sit up in a chair, roll over in bed, and assist with transfer to and from her wheelchair. ("Stroke Patient Increases Mobility with Aquatic Therapy," HydroWorx, July 12, 2013).

I found several other studies that showed there are significant benefits using aquatic therapy after a stroke. In a 2008 study two groups of stroke survivors were compared. One group received conventional physical therapy, the other aquatic therapy. The findings were that the aquatic group improved significantly more in strength, balance, and knee flexor strength than the conventional physical therapy group. (study by Dong Koog Noh et. al., Seoul National University College of Medicine, 2008).

Christine Shidla, Director of Wellness, Summit Place Senior Campus in Eden Prairie, Minnesota states, "For stroke survivors, we see at our facility, exercise in the water has the power to change their lives. Often our clients have been discharged from the hospital or land-based therapy because they have ceased to make gains. Undaunted and determined, they turn to us to develop innovative exercise programs in our underwater treadmill therapy pool. The results normally lead them to accomplish goals they could not otherwise achieve."

Finding an Aquatic Therapy Program and Facility:

Finding a facility is easy. Finding a facility close to your home that your insurance will cover can be more difficult. My advice is to do your own research by using the following resources:

Ask your therapist or the therapists at rehabilitation hospitals if they have a program or if they know of one nearby.

Check with your nearest YMCA as many have started aquatic therapy programs. (www.ymca. org to find programs and locations).

Use a computer search to find "aquatic therapy near you." Scroll down to aquatic therapy. Type in your zip code.

Contact Easter Seals at (1-800-221-6827). Many Easter Seals locations provide aquatic therapy.

Chapter 13: Risk Factors for Stroke *

"To some education is a bore; to most education is food for the brain and enrichment for the present and future" Ann Monnar (author)

Chances are that most readers of this chapter have had a stroke. The risk factors in this chapter, one or more of which may have contributed to your stroke, carry the same risk factors in preventing a second stroke. Risk factors are different than causes. There are two basic causes of a stroke. First, is the formation of a clot that makes its way to an artery that blocks blood flow to the brain. This causes what we know as an *Ischemic Stroke.* The second cause, a result of bleeding in the brain, is a *Hemorrhagic Stroke.* (Approximately 87% of strokes are ischemic; 13% are hemorrhagic).

Most stroke survivors and even the general public know the primary risk factors for stroke. These include high blood pressure, high cholesterol, diabetes, smoking, and family history. This chapter will look at all of these risk factors and secondary factors, some of which are too often overlooked.

High Blood Pressure: High blood pressure is the greatest risk factor for stroke. High BP puts unnecessary stress on blood vessels and arteries causing them to thicken and deteriorate. When blood vessel walls thicken, substances such as cholesterol may break off and block an artery to the brain causing an ischemic stroke. High blood pressure can also put undue stress on a vessel or artery leading to a brain bleed and a hemorrhagic stroke.

High LDL Cholesterol: High cholesterol, which causes plaque build-up, can block normal blood flow to the brain and cause an ischemic stroke.

Atherosclerosis is the progressive build-up of cholesterol or other fatty deposits in the arteries that will eventually block flow to the brain potentially causing a stroke.

<u>Peripheral Arterial Disease (PAD)</u>: When plaque build-up from cholesterol clogs the arteries, it can also lead to the blockage of blood supply to the legs. This causes leg cramps and should be a warning that you may have atherosclerosis in other arteries.

<u>Diabetes:</u> Diabetes causes destructive changes in the blood vessels throughout the body, including the brain. Over time, high glucose levels damage nerve and blood vessels, leading to complications including stroke. The health risk of cardiovascular disease, including stroke, is two and a half times greater in people with diabetes compared to people without diabetes. Further, stroke is the leading cause of death among people with diabetes.

<u>Smoking:</u> The risk of stroke for smokers is between two and two and a half times that of non smokers. Studies have shown that smoking reduces the amount of oxygen in the blood causing the heart to work harder and allowing blood clots to form more easily. Smoking also increases the amount of plaque in the arteries, which may block blood flow to the brain, causing a stroke.

<u>Atrial Fibrillation:</u> A person with A-Fib is five times more likely to have a stroke than someone without A-FIB. A-Fib is caused when the two upper chambers of the heart beat rapidly and unpredictably, producing irregular heartbeat. A-Fib is a risk for stroke because it allows blood to pool in the heart. This tends to form clots which can be carried to the brain, causing a stroke.

<u>Obstructive Sleep Apnea:</u>   Obstructive Sleep Apnea is more dangerous for men than women. This may be because more men suffer from the disorder and almost always at a younger age than women. Overall, sleep apnea doubles the risk of stroke. The risk increases with the severity of the disorder. Sleep Apnea is a sleep condition which includes loud snoring and breathing that stops and starts during sleep. The result is an interruption in breathing up to ten seconds and sometimes even more. This in turn decreases blood flow to the brain and can elevate blood pressure within the brain causing a possible hemorrhagic stroke. Obstructive Sleep Apnea can cause a whole host of health problems including A-Fib,

high blood pressure, and diabetes, all of which are risk factors for stroke. Doctors and hospitals now have home testing devices for Obstructive Sleep Apnea.

Alcohol Abuse: Healthcare professionals can give no definite reason why drinking alcohol in excess may increase the risk of stroke, but scientists and healthcare professionals agree that drinking more than two drinks a day increases the risk of stroke. It is thought that alcohol contributes to thinning of the blood vessels and decreases efficiency of heart function which can cause a hemorrhagic stroke and/or clot formation.

Carotid Artery Disease: The carotid arteries are located in both sides of the neck. They supply blood to the brain, so when one side or both are clogged by a clot, an ischemic stroke will surely occur. Avoid other ischemic stroke risks such as obesity and smoking to lower risk of CAD. CAD is usually diagnosed by a doctor using a stethoscope to hear blood flow on both sides of the neck.

Oral Contraceptives: Oral contraceptives nearly double the risk of stroke in women. Add obesity and smoking and the risk is much greater. I have mentored two women, one under forty, and one under thirty, who have had strokes that were attributed in part to oral contraceptives. How oral contraceptives can cause a stroke is not completely understood. Birth control pills now in use contain lower levels of estrogen than older versions. This has decreased the risk; however, risk factors should be discussed with the prescribing doctor.

Obesity and Belly Fat: In September, 2010, I wrote an article for strokenetwork.org explaining the relationship between obesity and stroke. The studies that I quoted conclude that the correlation between increasing stroke incidence and increasing degree of obesity was apparent independent of other risk factors. Further, people with bigger waist circumference (belly fat) are at even greater risk.

Prior Stroke, TIA, or Heart Attack: All of these increase the risk for stroke so it is important to be under the care of both a primary care physician and a neurologist. A TIA or Transient Ischemic Attack is a mini stroke caused by the same risk factors as a stroke. Chapter 14 explains the risk for stroke after having a TIA. People who have had a prior stroke are at risk of having a second stroke if the risk factors causing the first stroke are not eliminated.

Lipoprotein A, Homocystenes, and C Reactive Proteins: There is increasing evidence that high levels of these are risk factors for stroke. When getting a simple blood test (CBC), doctors seldom include these three. Ask your doctor to include these for your next CBC.

Arteriovenous Malformation and Cerebral Aneurism: Malformation in the cerebral arteries, such as an AVM or an aneurism, can cause a vein to burst causing a hemorrhagic stroke.

The following sources were used in writing this chapter:
National Stroke Association: www.stroke.org
American Heart Association: www.americanheart.org
Science Daily: www.sciencedaily.com
The National Institute of Health: www.nih.gov
www.answers.com

---

* This chapter was published in my earlier book, Brain Injury: Living a Productive Life after a Stroke or Traumatic Brain Injury.

Chapter 14: Transient Ischemic Attack *

"My dull brain was wrought with things forgotten" William Shakespeare

Almost everyone who has had a stroke knows what a TIA is. A Transient Ischemic Attack, sometimes called a mini-stroke, occurs when a clot blocks blood flow and oxygen to the brain just as a stroke will do. The difference is in the length of time that the blockage is in place. In a TIA, the clot clears itself so that the stroke-like symptoms of the blockage are temporary and therefore, damage to the brain is minimal or nonexistent.

Although the symptoms of TIA, such as numbness on one side of the face or body, blurred vision, slurred speech, dizziness, etc., usually last only for a short time, sometimes less than ten minutes, the TIA should be taken seriously. Studies have shown that patients are at risk of having a stroke after a TIA with the greatest risk coming within the first three days, and that between 24% and 29% of patients who experience a TIA will have a stroke within five years if not treated.

Research suggests that between 500,000 and 600,000 strokes occur each year and approximately 10% of strokes are preceded by TIAs. Dr. S. Claiborne Johnston, Professor of Neurology at the University of California, San Francisco, stated at the 25th International Stroke Conference that "the acronym TIA should stand for Take Action Immediately." The symptoms of TIA often are not taken seriously by patients and physicians alike because they are usually short-lived and often mild. However, Dr. Johnston states, "TIAs are very, very, ominous." **

Betty Collins, a Registered Nurse and Facilitator of a support group at Kessler Institute in West Orange, New Jersey, concurs. She states, "I think many people just hope it goes away and when it does, they don't think about it again; even to the point of not mentioning it to their physicians." She adds that, "It is difficult for doctors to order a range of tests when symptoms are no longer present and a rationale for each test must be given for insurance purposes."

I interviewed Dr. Sean Savitz, a neurologist at the University of Texas Medical Center in Houston, by telephone because I wanted to get first hand a doctor's perspective on TIAs. He emphasized that it is very important to seek medical treatment for a TIA to ascertain the patient's risk factors for a stroke such as high blood pressure and diabetes. TIAs have different symptoms for different patients. Some TIAs result in drooping features on one side of the face, blurred vision in an eye, or tingling on one side of the body. Thus, people are not sure if they need treatment because they may not identify their particular symptoms as TIAs.

If you experience what you think might be a TIA, you should call for emergency medical service for immediate transport to a hospital equipped to care for people with stroke and TIA. A PSC (Primary Stroke Center) is best. Never attempt to drive yourself to the hospital nor should you have a friend or relative drive you. If a medical complication occurs on the way to the hospital, EMS personnel are best trained to respond.

Diagnosis: Once the patient reaches the Primary Stroke Center or hospital, a complete neurological exam is called for. This may include:

The standard Mini-Mental Status Exam to observe the patient's attentiveness, interaction with the examiner, language use, memory skills, etc.

A CT scan to identify any bleeding or mass that may be causing the symptoms.

An MRI (magnetic resonance imagery) to examine areas of the brain affected by the TIA.

An MRA (magnetic resonance angiogram) and/or an ultrasound to detect blockages or plaque build-up in the blood vessels. Special attention is paid to the carotid artery. If blockage is detected, removing plaque by surgery may be necessary.

A check for heart problems using an echocardiogram or an electrocardiogram (ECG).

Treatment: The treatment, of course, is determined after the results of the above mentioned tests are complete. Treatments vary from patient to patient. Since the goal is to prevent a stroke from occurring, great attention is paid to treat medical problems including high blood pressure, high cholesterol, smoking, and diabetes, which may have been the cause of the TIA in the first place. Other treatments include:

a. Anti-platelet therapy, to reduce the risk of platelet clumping and new clot formation. Dr.Nina Solinsky, of the University of Virginia Health Center states, "Aspirin is the most powerful anti-platelet drug available."

b. Other drugs may be added, such as dipyridamole (Persantine) if need be.

c. Anti-coagulant therapy is designed to decrease the risk of blood clots forming in the arteries. The most common of these medications is warfarin (Coumadin). This type of medication is generally prescribed for patients who have had previous TIAs or are otherwise at high risk for a stroke.

d. Each year, about 240,000 people in the U.S. are diagnosed with a TIA. Recognize the symptoms so if it happens to you, you can take action. Call 911 immediately. It may save your life or prevent a life of disability.

---

* This chapter was published in my earlier book, <u>Brain Injury: Living a Productive Life after a stroke or Traumatic Brain Injury.</u>

** This information comes from an article in FAMILY PRACTICE NEWS, April 15, 2000, by Eric Goldman.

Chapter 15: Is Chiropractic Neck Manipulation a Significant Cause of Stroke?

Into each life some rain must fall" Henry Wadsworth Longfellow

I had never heard of any relationship between chiropractic neck manipulation and stroke until a few years ago. Even then, I did not give it a second thought. I have been going to chiropractors since I hurt my back in college some 45 years ago. I had always asked the chiropractor to manipulate my back, but not my neck because I had no neck pain and the few times that I had my neck manipulated, I did not like the way it felt.

Recently, I happened to see articles about a relationship between chiropractic neck manipulation and stroke. When I decided to research this subject, I was surprised that so many articles and studies had been done on the issue.

The vulnerable artery in the neck is called the vertebral artery. Due to the position of this artery, sudden neck manipulation could stretch it and rupture its lining causing a brain bleed which in turn causes a blood clot to form over the injured area. This clot may subsequently be dislodged and block a smaller artery that supplies blood to the brain causing a stroke. (Norris, JW and others. "Sudden Neck Movement and Cervical Artery Dissection." Canadian Medical Journal 163:38-40, 2000.)

I have read many articles and studies and have found many contradictions, especially between studies done by chiropractors and chiropractic organizations and the studies done by other researchers. What was most striking to me was that various researchers speculate that the risk of having a stroke after chiropractic neck manipulation falls between 1 in 30,000 and 1in 10 million. The reason for this discrepancy is twofold:

It is difficult to know if a patient who has a stroke sometime after chiropractic manipulation had a stroke because of that manipulation, or whether there was a weakness or dissection (tear) in the artery before chiropractic treatment.

When a patient has a stroke, it is rare for the neurologist to ask if the patient had had chiropractic manipulation. Even in a clinical study, it is difficult to draw conclusions because there is no way to tell if a patient would have had a stroke anyway.

To clarify things, I have decided to summarize studies involving both researchers not connected with chiropractics and studies where chiropractors were involved.

Study: Researchers at Stanford Stroke Center conducted a study sponsored by the American Heart Association. 177 neurologists out of 486 (just over 1/3) responded to the question, "How many patients have you seen in the last two years who suffered a stroke within 24 hours of chiropractic neck manipulation. The number was 56. One might conclude that the number would be approximately 160 if all 486 had responded. This was in California which had 19% of the nation's chiropractors in 1991. Lee, K.P., and others. "Neurological Complications Following Chiropractic Manipulation: a Survey of California Neurologists." Neurology 45: 1213-1215, 1995.

Study: Researchers at the Canadian Stroke Consortium studied 98 cases in which external trauma, ranging from trivial to severe, was identified as the trigger for strokes caused by blood clots formed in arteries to the brain. The researchers concluded that 38 of these stroke cases were apparently caused by chiropractic neck manipulation. (Beletsky V. "Chiropractic Neck Manipulation May be Underestimated as a Cause of Stroke." Presented at the American Stroke Association 27th International Stroke Conference, San Antonio, Texas, February, 2002).

Study: A study was conducted using records from 1993 - 2002 from Ontario, Canada hospitals to compare Vertebral Stroke survivors that were treated by a chiropractor versus those treated by a primary care physician prior to a stroke. The study concluded that although there is an association between chiropractic care and Vertebral Strokes there is a similar association between

Vertebral Strokes and primary care treatment by their PCP. The study suggests that an undiagnosed vertebral artery dissection (a tear in the artery wall which results in a blood clot) was present prior to treatment. In other words, the stroke would have occurred regardless of treatment. (J. David Cassidy, DC and others. "Risk of Vertebrobasilar stroke and Chiropractic Care." Spine. 33(4S):176-S183, 2008).

Study: In a 2007 study 377 members of the British and Scottish Chiropractic Associations and 19,000 patients were asked whether complications occurred after chiropractic neck manipulations. No strokes were reported and only mild side effects were reported, such as headaches or dizziness in a very small percentage of those questioned (less than 5%). Researchers concluded that the risk for stroke after neck manipulation is low to very low. (Thiel HW and others. "Safety of Chiropractic Manipulation of the Spine." Spine 32:2375-2378, 2007).

Conclusions: These conclusions are mine based on all of the research that I have read.

1. There is evidence that there is an association between chiropractic neck manipulation and vertebral artery stroke. However, the risk is very small.

2. Chiropractors should inform patients of the minimal risk similar to cautions given in TV ads about risk factors and side effects when taking a medication.

3. There is no conclusive evidence that chiropractic neck manipulation relieves headaches or neck pain, so it might be better to limit your treatment to spinal manipulation. Ask your chiropractor if neck manipulation is necessary to treat your particular problem.

4. Children should avoid chiropractic neck manipulation.

5. Despite all of the studies concerning the relationship between chiropractic manipulation and Vertebral Artery Stroke (Vertebrobasilar Stroke), there is no satisfactory conclusive evidence to determine this issue.

Part III: Amazing Stroke Stories

Chapter 16: Jean-Dominique Bauby

"No one feels your empty stomach, but everyone does your empty brain"
M. F. Moonzajer (author)

Many have heard about Jean-Dominique Bauby (Jean-Do to those closest to him) from his book and the film adaptation <u>The Diving Bell and the Butterfly.</u> The title came from Bauby himself from the notion that while his body was submerged (like a diving bell) and it was impossible to move, his mind, imagination, and memory were free and as light as a butterfly's wings.

In December, 1995, at the age of 43, Bauby suffered a massive stroke while being driven by his chauffer in the country to pick up his son Theophile. He was in a coma for three weeks and when he woke, he could not move any part of his body including his head and mouth, except his left eyelid. The condition is called locked-in syndrome. (More about locked-in-syndrome later).

Jean-Dominique was the editor-in-chief of French Elle magazine. He had a ten year live-in relationship with Sylvie De La Rochefoucauld, the mother of his children, Theophile and Celeste. Two years before his stroke, he moved out of the house and was in a relationship with Florence Ben Sadoun, a film, fashion, and beauty journalist for Elle magazine.

The film is award winning but has several differences from the factual book. The main difference is that his girlfriend, Florence Ben Sadoun was by his side during the two years of his hospitalization. She would take the three hour drive two to three times per week. She was by his side when he died in 1997 from complications from infection and pneumonia. The mother of his children, Sylvie De La Rochefoucauld (they were never married as the film portrays) was long estranged from Bauby and rarely visited him in the hospital. (The film has Sylvie as the devoted partner). She was in New York with her boyfriend at the time he died.

While in the hospital, Bauby made only marginal improvement but began his memoir with the help of his nurse/ghost writer, his speech therapist, and Florence. Letters of the alphabet were dictated to him and he would blink when the letter he wanted was said. This was a painstaking, time consuming project that took an estimated 200,000 blinks to complete The Diving Bell and the Butterfly. The book was published in 1997 just before Bauby died.

The cast of characters in Jean-Dominique Bauby's life:

Sylvie De La Rochefoucauld – Sylvie was in a ten year relationship with Bauby and they lived together in a Paris suburb in a luxurious house complete with swimming pool and tennis court. They had two children together: a boy named Theophile and a girl named Celeste. Although the film portrays her as the grieving wife, she had moved on with her life and rarely visited Jean-Dominique in the hospital. At the time of this writing she is the managing director of Zero Virgule Deaux, a public relations firm outside Paris, France. She is 63 years old. No further information could be obtained.

Florence Ben Sadoun – Florence was in a two year relationship with Bauby before his stroke and stuck with him until he died. She was a frequent companion to Bauby while he was in the hospital. After his death, she continued to raise her two children from a previous marriage and continued her career as a journalist. In 2001 she published a novel, The False Widow. In 2008 she became the managing editor of She magazine and currently is that magazine's deputy chief editor. She is married to actor Gillis-Gaston Dreyfus. She is 53 years old.

Sandrine Fichou – Sandrine became Bauby's speech therapist and when it was discovered that he could communicate by blinking his left eye, she devised an "alphabet of silence." Letters could be dictated in the order of those most often used, allowing him to blink when he heard the correct letter. Letters became words and words became sentences. Sangrine did not like the movie because, "it was not like that in real life." In the film, Bauby is heard telling her that he wanted to die. Sandrine states, "He never said that." There is no up to date information about Sandrine because she has declined all interviews and she demands privacy.

Claude Mendibil – When it became known that Bauby wanted to write his memoirs using Sangrine Fichou's "silent alphabet," publisher Robert Lafont sent the experienced ghost writer and freelance book editor Claude Mendibil to take on the job. The now 58 year old took an apartment near the hospital so that she could go daily to transcribe Bauby's thoughts. She spent two months on the project and the result was a best seller, <u>The Diving Bell and the Butterfly</u>. Claude, never married, has a daughter Raphaelle and lives in Paris opposite the cemetery where Jean-Dominique is buried. She visits his grave often.

Theophile and Celeste Bauby – Jean-Dominique's children were eleven (Theo) and nine (Celeste). They are 30 and 28 respectively at the time of this writing. After Bauby's death, their mother Sylvie raised them alone. In 2008 they both commented on the film and both said it was difficult to watch their father in that condition. To the best of my knowledge, it is the last time either Theophile or Celeste was interviewed.

Locked-In Syndrome:

The condition of Jean-Dominique Bauby after his stroke is typical of one who suffers from locked-in syndrome. Nearly all muscles from head to toe are paralyzed except for the eyes. This means the patient cannot talk or move any part of his body.

Causes of LIS include traumatic brain injury, stroke, amyotrophic lateral disease (ALS or Lou Gehrig's disease), in some cases, Multiple Sclerosis, and medication overdose. There is no treatment for LIS and 90% of patients die within the first four months.

Sources:

"Blink of an Eye," Karen S. Schneider, People Magazine, June 2, 1997.

"Obituary: Jean-Dominique Bauby," James Kirkup, The Independent, March 12, 1997.

"A Story Told in the Blink of an Eye," Elizabeth Day, The Guardian, January 6, 2008.

"The Real Love Story Behind the Diving Bell and the Butterfly," Janine DiGiovanni, <u>The Guardian,</u> November 29, 2008.

"The Truth About The Diving Bell and The Butterfly," Beth Arnold, <u>Salon Media Group</u>, February 23, 2008.

Chapter 17: Woodrow Wilson

"As you fulfill your emotions, your brain will change and form new patterns, which is the goal" Deepak Chopra

Woodrow Wilson was the 28th President of the United States, serving from 1913 through January, 1921. If you read a biography about him, it is likely that you will read about the severe stroke that he had in October of 1919. Many historians, however, believe he had several strokes and transient Ischemic Accidents (mini strokes) well before 1919.

In 1896, at age 30, it is believed that Wilson suffered his first stroke while a professor at Princeton University. This left brain stroke weakened his right hand and arm. In time, his condition improved so that he could resume normal life.

In 1904 and 1906, he suffered two more left brain strokes while President of Princeton University, which again weakened his right arm and affected his vision. These strokes suggest that he was prone to blood clots which we can easily treat with medications today. Despite his condition, which also included severe periodic headaches, his career advanced as he was elected governor of New Jersey in 1910, and was elected President in 1912.

The United States entered World War I in 1917. When it ended in 1919 and after the Treaty of Versailles was signed, officially ending the war, it needed to be ratified by each nation's government. Wilson had been successful in convincing the other signees that a League of Nations (a prelude to the United Nations), an organization to prevent further wars, was necessary and it became part of the treaty.

But conservative Senators blocked the ratification of the treaty, so Wilson decided to take his cause directly to the people. He ventured on a country wide tour across America by train, speaking at town meetings all across his route.

The train left Washington D.C. on September 3rd but by September 26th, Wilson was exhausted and his heath was deteriorating. The train headed back to Washington where Wilson did his best to rest.

On October 2, 1919, the President's wife, Edith Wilson, found her husband on the bathroom floor. The President had suffered a massive stroke. He was paralyzed on the right side and his vision was impaired. With two doctors to treat him, Dr. Grayson, the President's physician, and Dr. Ruffin, Mrs. Wilson's private physician, Wilson was stabilized. The doctors and Mrs. Wilson formed a shield between her husband and the outside world and for the next seventeen months, the President was mostly bed ridden and all communication with President Wilson went through Mrs. Wilson. He finished his term without the public ever knowing of their President's condition.

Woodrow Wilson's term effectively ended with the Presidential election of 1920. Many historians label the period after Wilson's stroke by calling Edith Wilson the first woman President.

Although his health gradually improved, he never really recovered. In 1924, five years after retirement, Wilson suffered another massive stroke, this time fatal.

Two points are important. First, despite the strokes that Woodrow Wilson suffered, without the clinical rehabilitation methods or the preventative medications of today, he was able to accomplish a great deal including two presidential terms. Second, with the news media today, both print media and television, it would be impossible to keep a president's severe condition a secret from the general public.

Sources:
"President Woodrow Wilson Overcomes Stroke and Leads a Country," Stroke for Dummies, John R. Marler, M.D., Chapter 19, pp. 317-318, 2005.

"President Wilson Suffers a Stroke," Eyewitness to History.com, January 28, 2014.

Chapter 18: Dan Reichert

Every now and then a man's mind is stretched by a new idea or sensation, and never shrinks back to its former dimensions" Oliver Wendell Holmes

Dan Reichert is a legend around Wayne, Pennsylvania. The 80 year old former Navy Seal had been coaching at the Martin's Dam Swim Club since the 1960's but has recently retired from coaching. Many of his former swimmers, including a teenage Olympian, are a bit surprised by his announcement. Many have expressed the fact that they cannot imagine being at the pool without him.

Dan grew up in Brooklyn, New York, and went to Midwood High School. After high school he joined the Navy, eventually becoming a Navy Seal. In high school, swimming was merely an afterthought. He played football in the fall and baseball in the spring, but was idle in the winter. He explained, "My father excused me from chores if I played a sport so I opted for the swim team."

After high school and the Navy, Dan got a job with a diving company as a diver and salesman, and he started coaching at the local YMCA. He realized that he loved coaching so he decided to get a teaching degree so he could coach on the high school level.

Dan decided to go to West Chester Teachers College (now West Chester University) in Pennsylvania where he received a degree in physical education. He soon became a teacher and taught physical education and coached swimming in the Upper Darby and Radnor school districts before going to Conestoga High School where he taught physical education and started the swim team. He remained at Conestoga for 21 years until his retirement. After he stepped down from Conestoga, he coached only club teams until he was persuaded to become assistant coach at West Chester East High School under head coach Craig Erb. Two years later Erb stepped down and Dan became a head coach once again.

Besides high school, Dan's coaching career includes 16 summers at Upper Main Line YMCA, stints at Suburban Swim Center in Newtown Square, Newtown, Pennsylvania, Westtown Aquatic, in Westtown, Pennsylvania, 16 years at Immaculata College, where his wife Lynn was Athletic Director, and summers at Martin's Dam for more than 45 years.

In January, 2011, Dan was home and suddenly found himself on the floor. He could not speak and could not move. He was flown by helicopter to Jefferson University Hospital. "It was a severe stroke," said Pascal Jabbour, Director of the Division of Neurovascular Surgery at Jefferson. "His life was at risk. He wasn't moving the right side of his body and he couldn't talk or understand." He spent his rehab at Bryn Mawr Rehab facility and he worked hard. His spirits were always high and he never doubted that he would recover. That summer, four months after the stroke, he was back at Martin's Dam helping the new coaches.

Dan has always loved coaching and his swimmers love him. Four of his charges at West Chester East, Kelly Nelson, Caitlin Meehan, Erin Meehan, and Meredith Chapla, were all high school all-Americans and college swimmers. They all also have great memories of their coach. "Danny is one of the great people any of us has known," Caitlin Meehan said. "You want to swim well for him more than for yourself." Kelly Nelson states, "He's like a grandpop. Words cannot describe him. He does everything." Erin Meehan remembered, "You can't ask for anything more in a coach. He supported me through everything and has been so understanding. We had so much fun with him."

The summer after the stroke, using a walker for balance, Dan came back to Martin's Dam to help his former pupil Philip Munger, now a coach at Martin's Falls. The thousands of swimmers that he has coached include Munger, now 27, and his mother, Dorothy Munger. "I first met Dan when I was ten years old and I'm 62 now. Can you imagine coming out of the Navy Seals and working with ten year old girls?"

Dan Reichert retired from coaching at age 80. Martin's Dam honored him in 2013. Scores of his former swimmers came to say good-bye. Dan's remarkable recovery should be an inspiration to others.

Sources:

"Swim Coach Dan Reichert, 80, Triumphing Over Stroke," Paul Jablow, Philadelphia Inquirer, August 4, 2013.

"Recovering From a Stroke," Josh Goldstein, Jefferson University Newsletter, August 5, 2013.

"Vikings' Swim Coach is one Proud Mentor. Dan Reichert Loves his Job," Ira Josephs, Philadelphia Inquirer, March 27, 2005.

"Dan Reichert Stays in the Swim of Things," Dan Beideman, Philadelphia Inquirer, February 22, 2006.

Chapter 19: Jackie Mayer

"Life is really simple but we insist on making it complicated" Confucius

Jackie Mayer was born in Sandusky, Ohio in 1943. She won the Miss Ohio beauty contest while a freshman at Northwestern University and left college after one year to tour as a singer with bandleader Fred Waring's Pennsylvanians band. Then, in 1963, at the suggestion of a friend, she entered the Miss America contest. She was crowned the winner at the Atlantic City Convention Hall in front of 30,000 people. It was a dream come true and fortune seemed to follow Jackie.

The year after she was crowned Miss America, Jackie was busy fulfilling Miss America obligations with speaking events and social engagements. Later in 1963, she became engaged to

John Townsend, a racing executive. They were married in 1964 and had two children, a son Billy and a daughter Kelly. During this time, Jackie completed her studies at Northwestern University earning a degree in Speech.

Fast forward to 1970. When Jackie was 28 years old, after celebrating Thanksgiving with family and friends, she was awakened in the early morning by the cries of her nine month old daughter. She found herself unable to get up and unable to speak. Jackie had had a massive, life threatening stroke. She had complained of headaches most of Thanksgiving Day and had retired to bed early. She could not move her right side and struggled to wake her husband John for help.

Jackie was rushed to the hospital and fought for her life. She survived and began a seven year recovery process. She received an out-of-court settlement with Ortho Pharmaceutical, manufacturers of the birth control pills that doctors blamed for the stroke.

Through the help and emotional support of her family and friends, Jackie gained back motor and verbal skills. Her husband John came to the hospital twice every day and later at home, her young son became her teacher. Gradually, she began to walk, learned to speak, read, and write, and regained most of what the stroke had taken away.

After her recovery, she became a motivational speaker and a spokeswoman for the National Heart and Stroke Association. Jackie appeared on multiple talk shows and has been featured in many national magazines. Today, at age 72 (at the time of this writing) she still lectures to corporations, healthcare organizations, charity organizations such as Rotary Clubs, and other major events. She has won numerous awards and has been given two honorary doctorate degrees.

Traveling around the country for over 30 years, her message is pretty much the same. Understanding the risk factors for and recognizing the signs of a stroke are important for everyone to know. She tells her life story and tells everyone that no matter what troubles they may have, or illnesses that occur, to always keep a positive attitude and work to improve yourself. She usually ends her talk by reading the poem, "Oh God, Forgive me When I Whine."

Sources:

"A Former Miss America Tells of Her Crowning Achievement: Recovery From a Stroke," Jacqueline Mayer Towsend, People.com, May 17, 1982.

"There She Is, Miss America," Beverly Lane Lorenz, Carolina Gateway (S.C.), January 9, 2014.

"The Jackie Mayer Story," jackiemayer.com, 2013.

Chapter 20: George Frideric Handel

The mind does most of its best thinking when we are not there. The answers are there in the morning" Alain de Botton (Swiss-British author)

George Frideric Handel was born in 1685 in Halle, Germany. He grew up and was educated there until he moved to Hamburg, Germany, at the age of 18. There he began his career as a violinist for the Hamburg Opera. He loved music and was exposed early to German church music, but in Hamburg he quickly found opera and ballet. He was educated and intelligent and spoke English, German, French, and Italian.

His first major musical composition failed, but before he reached the age of 20, he produced two successful operas. In the following years he lived in Rome, Florence, and Venice where he studied and composed. He later moved to England where his fame as a composer grew. In 1714, he wrote Water Music, a collection of orchestral movements often published in three movements, or keys. It is usually performed by large orchestras and is popular at outdoor performances. Water Music brought considerable fortune and fame to the still young composer.

In the years that followed, Handel started three commercial opera companies in London to supply the English nobility with Italian opera. From 1715 to 1737, he wrote many operas and other compositions making him one of the most famous people in England.

In 1937, at the age of 52, Handel suffered a stroke. His right hand and arm became useless. He left England to recover in Aachen, Germany, and also visited France during this period of recovery. He lived a secluded life in Germany where he recovered but continued to suffer from depression.

He returned to England in 1740 where he wrote several choral compositions. A re-charged Handel wrote his most famous work, Messiah, in 1741, in just three weeks. He suffered a second stroke in 1752, which left him blind in one eye. Despite his hardships, he continued to write music until his death in 1759. He is buried in Westminster Abbey in London.

Sources:

"The Case of George Frideric Handel," New England Journal of Medicine, September, 1989.

"Composer George Frideric Handel Writes Messiah After Stroke", John R. Marler, M.D., Stroke For Dummies, 2005.

Appendix I: Helpful web-sites

This list includes web-sites published in my previous book with many additions.

Web-sites

www.americanheart.org

www.nih.gov

www.ninds.nih.gov

www.clinicaltrials.gov

www.curebraindisease.org

www.strokeassociation.org

www.nationalstrokeassociation.org

www.strokesafe.org

www.safestroke.org

www.biaa.org

www.stroke.org

www.aan.com/patients (neurology)

www.thefamilycaregiver.org

www.aphasia.org

www.aphasia.net

www.asha.org (for aphasia)
www.academyofaphasia.org
www.apraxia-kids.org
www.alexiafoundation.org
www.wellspouse.org
www.dailystrength.org
www.caringbridge.org

The following is a web-site list of resources concerning clinical trials.
www.acurian.com
www.centerwatch.com
www.clinicaltrials.gov
www.rehabtrials.org
www.cc.nih.gov/recruit/index.html

Appendix II: Brain Injury: Living a Productive Life After a Stroke or Traumatic Brain Injury The following is the Table of Contents of my first book published in October, 2013.

About the Author:

Walter Kilcullen is a retired guidance counselor from Morris Knolls High School, Denville, New Jersey. He has been a mentor for stroke and traumatic brain injury survivors for the past 14 years. He is also a staff writer for strokenetwork.org.

He published his first book, *Brain Injury: Living a Productive Life After a Stroke or Traumatic Brain Injury* in October, 2013.

He resides in Allamuchy, New Jersey with his wife. You can reach Walter at harmony29@verizon.net.